Fibromyalgia For Dummies®

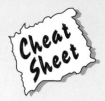

Cheat Sheet

KT-557-691

Getting Enough Sleep

Constant insomnia won't cause fibromyalgia, but it can worsen or trigger a major flare-up. Get at least seven hours of sleep every night. Here are some tips to make sure sleep happens:

- Don't eat or drink caffeinated foods or beverages after 8 p.m. — they can keep you awake. In fact, not eating at all after 8 p.m. is best.
- Make sure your bed is comfortable.
- If a snoring partner keeps you awake at night, make him or her seek help.
- Save your bedroom for sleep and sex only. Don't watch TV in bed or work on papers you've brought home from the office.
- Ask your doctor about sleep medications if nothing else works.

Avoiding Trigger Foods

No food can create fibromyalgia in a person who doesn't already have it, but some foods can make the condition worse. Try to avoid the following foods and beverages, which can worsen your symptoms:

- Anything with lots of caffeine (colas, chocolate, tea, and coffee)
- Foods containing MSG (monosodium glutamate, a flavoring) such as frozen pizza or corn chips
- Alcoholic beverages

Dealing with Doubters

Some people out there still think that fibromyalgia is not a real illness or that it's a diagnosis your doctor gives you if she can't think of anything else and wants to assign some name to your symptoms. These folks are wrong. Fibromyalgia is a very real and painful medical problem. So, what do you say to the doubters out there?

- Pain studies have shown that people with fibromyalgia experience pain faster and more intensely.
- Studies have shown that people with fibromyalgia have abnormal levels of stress hormones and other biochemicals. Researchers don't know yet if the increased presence of these biochemicals is the cause of fibromyalgia, but it's a clear indicator of a problem.
- People used to think depression was fake too, and now, most people know better. Fibromyalgia is just as real.
- Most people with fibromyalgia are women, and some people think all women's problems are exaggerated. It took awhile for people to catch up to the reality of migraines and premenstrual syndrome.

For Dummies: Bestselling Book Series for Beginners

Fibromyalgia For Dummies®

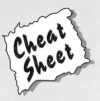

Communicating with Your Doc

Most of the time when you have fibromyalgia, your doctor will ask you the right questions that lead him or her to the right diagnosis. But to be on the safe side, if your doctor doesn't ask, make sure you volunteer information regarding any of these symptoms or events that apply to you:

- Morning stiffness (a common problem for people with fibromyalgia)
- Frequent or constant trouble sleeping
- Extreme fatigue that occurs day after day, even when you haven't done anything
- Pain that changes intensity (sometimes severe; other times more moderate)
- Recent physical trauma (a car crash, for example)
- Family members diagnosed with fibromyalgia (especially a parent or a sibling)

Coping with the Pain Effectively

Many people need medications, either over-the-counter or prescribed drugs, to help them cope with the pain from their fibromyalgia. But other methods are proven to decrease pain, and they may work for you. Consider trying one (or all) of these choices:

- Massage therapy
- Regular aerobic exercise
- Relaxation therapy
- Acupuncture treatments
- Icing or heating the painful areas
- Botox injections

Copyright © 2002 Wiley Publishing, Inc.
All rights reserved.

Item 5441-7.

For more information about Wiley Publishing,
call 1-800-762-2974.

For Dummies: Bestselling Book Series for Beginners

About the Authors

Roland Staud, MD is a rheumatologist and an associate professor of medicine at the University of Florida in Gainesville, Florida, and a noted and internationally admired medical researcher. Dr. Staud's cutting-edge research on fibromyalgia for the National Institutes of Health and the Arthritis Foundation clearly demonstrated that patients with fibromyalgia syndrome (FMS) are more pain-sensitive and their pain lasts longer than for those without FMS.

At the American College of Rheumatology's Annual Scientific Meeting in 2000, Dr. Staud presented his research and pointed out that, "Our findings provide evidence for abnormal central nervous system mechanism of pain in fibromyalgia patients and have significant implications for future therapies, which need to target these abnormal pain mechanisms."

Dedicated to helping FMS patients by sharing his knowledge as much as possible, Dr. Staud is greatly appreciated by attendees at major national and international fibromyalgia and arthritis conferences, where he is a frequent speaker. He is also on the advisory board of *Fibromyalgia Awareness* magazine. In addition, he is a reviewer for the following medical publications: the *Journal of Clinical Rheumatology*, the *Journal of Pain,* and *Pain*. Dr. Staud has authored many medical journal articles on fibromyalgia and other topics.

Dr. Staud is a diplomate of the American Board of Rheumatology and the American Board of Internal Medicine. He is a member of the American College of Physicians, the American College of Rheumatology, the International Association for the Study of Pain, the American Pain Society, the International Myopain Society, the Florida Medical Association, and the Florida Society of Rheumatology. Dr. Staud is licensed to practice medicine in Florida and California.

Christine Adamec has been a freelance writer for more than 20 years, concentrating on self-help and medical/health issues. She has authored and coauthored 14 books, including *The Encyclopedia of Diabetes* (Facts On File, Inc.), *How to Stop Heartburn* (Wiley), and *Moms with ADD: A Self-Help Manual* (Taylor), as well as written numerous magazine and newspaper health features.

Ms. Adamec is a member of the American Medical Writers Association, the American Society of Journalists & Authors, and the Authors Guild.

Dedication

Dr. Staud would like to dedicate this book to all fibromyalgia volunteers who participated in his studies at the University of Florida, helping him to characterize the abnormal pain mechanisms of fibromyalgia syndrome.

Christine Adamec would like to dedicate this book to her ever-patient husband, John Adamec.

Acknowledgments

The authors would like to acknowledge the assistance of the following individuals: Esther Gwinnell, MD, an author and psychiatrist in private practice in Portland, Oregon and an associate clinical professor of psychiatry at Oregan Health and Science University; Joseph Kandel, MD, an author, a neurologist, the medical director of Neuroscience and Spine Associates in Naples, Florida, and associate clinical professor of Wright State University School of Medicine in Dayton, Ohio; and Alec Sohmer, Esq., an attorney from Brockton, Massachusetts, who assists people who have fibromyalgia and other medical problems with Social Security disability claims. In addition, the authors also thank Marie Mercer, reference librarian at the DeGroodt Public Library in Palm Bay, Florida, for her assistance in locating very hard-to-find journal articles on fibromyalgia. They would also like to thank the nearly 100 people with fibromyalgia who frankly and candidly responded to questions on how fibromyalgia has affected their lives and how they have coped with it.

The authors also especially thank their editor Alissa D. Schwipps, for her careful attention, advice, and positive feedback throughout this project.

Publisher's Acknowledgments

We're proud of this book; please send us your comments through our Dummies online registration form located at www.dummies.com/register/.

Some of the people who helped bring this book to market include the following:

Acquisitions, Editorial, and Media Development

Project Editor: Alissa D. Schwipps

Acquisitions Editor: Natasha Graf

Copy Editor: Chrissy Guthrie

Technical Editor: Jonathon Graf, M.D.

Editorial Manager: Jennifer Ehrlich

Editorial Assistant: Nívea C. Strickland

Cover Photo: © Rob Gage / Getty Images / FPG

Production

Project Coordinator: Nancee Reeves

Layout and Graphics: Scott Bristol, Amanda Carter, Joyce Haughey, LeAndra Johnson, Stephanie D. Jumper, Barry Offringa, Julie Trippetti, Jeremey Unger

Special Art: Kathryn Born, Medical Illustrator

Proofreader: John Greenough, Andy Hollandbeck, Angel Perez, TECHBOOKS Production Services

Indexer: TECHBOOKS Production Services

Special Help: Mike Baker, Ben Nussbaum Chad Sievers

Publishing and Editorial for Consumer Dummies

Diane Graves Steele, Vice President and Publisher, Consumer Dummies

Joyce Pepple, Acquisitions Director, Consumer Dummies

Kristin A. Cocks, Product Development Director, Consumer Dummies

Michael Spring, Vice President and Publisher, Travel

Brice Gosnell, Publishing Director, Travel

Suzanne Jannetta, Editorial Director, Travel

Publishing for Technology Dummies

Andy Cummings, Acquisitions Director

Composition Services

Gerry Fahey, Vice President of Production Services

Debbie Stailey, Director of Composition Services

Contents at a Glance

Table of Contents

Introduction

Fibromyalgia is a chronic medical problem that can sometimes be quite a daunting challenge to handle for the people who have it. But if you have fibromyalgia, you may find comfort in the fact that you're not alone. Fibromyalgia affects 6 million or more people in the United States and millions more in other countries. You can also find comfort in the fact that you can beat (or at least decrease) the problems that you and others are experiencing that stem from fibromyalgia.

Also known as fibromyalgia syndrome (FMS), fibromyalgia's major symptom is pain in the muscles and tendons throughout the body. (And for some people, the pain and its location can vary from day to day.) FMS pain often occurs without a specific cause or injury, sometimes long after trauma or infections.

Yet some people, including some doctors, persist in thinking that "fibromyalgia" is just another word for "hypochondria" — or maybe even "slacker" or "goof-off." They think that people who say they have fibromyalgia are really lazy or crazy — or both. They dismiss FMS as just another "disease of the month."

They're wrong. The pain isn't imaginary, and the problem is no fad. Studies that I've conducted at the University of Florida have proven that subjects diagnosed with fibromyalgia suffer heightened pain sensitivity, and they also retain pain longer than those individuals without the syndrome.

True, if fibromyalgia sufferers are depressed, anxious, or stressed, they'll feel worse. But, no, depression, anxiety, and stress don't actually *cause* fibromyalgia. People with FMS will have pain whether they're upset or not. But their pain often becomes greater when they're distressed.

What does fibromyalgia feel like? Many people say that to truly understand how FMS feels, think about what you feel like when you have the flu. Recall the aching and pain in parts of your body or in your entire body. Then, multiply those achy feelings by about 10 times. Now, imagine feeling that way *every day*. THAT is what fibromyalgia feels like for a lot of people. Pretty nasty.

The good news is that you can feel better with both the traditional and alternative medications and treatments as well as with the lifestyle choices that I describe in this book. They work for other people, and they can help you (or someone you know who suffers from FMS), too.

About This Book

I have two goals in writing this book. First, I want to show that fibromyalgia pain is real. This goal is important because some doubters are still out there. Second, I want to discuss the pain of FMS and provide current information on medications, alternative remedies, lifestyle changes, and other treatments that work.

You don't have to read this book from the first page straight on through to the end — although you certainly can if you want to. You may instead want to read my first chapter to get a feel and flavor for the rest of the book. Then you can use the table of contents at the front of the book or the index in the back to help you move on to the chapters that interest you the most.

Also, keep an eye out for the many personal stories that I've sprinkled throughout the book. They come from real people who suffer from fibromyalgia.

Conventions Used in This Book

The following conventions are used throughout the text to make things consistent and easy to understand:

- All Web addresses appear in `mono font`.
- New terms appear in *italics* and are closely followed by an easy-to-understand definition.
- **Bold** is used to highlight the action parts of numbered steps or keywords in bulleted lists.
- Sidebars, which are enclosed in a shaded gray box, include information that may fascinate you but that isn't critical to your understanding of FMS.

Also, you may have noticed that two names appear on the front cover, but I use the singular pronoun "I" in the text. I do so because this book reflects only my views as a medical professional, while Christine Adamec, an experienced medical writer, assists with the preparation and production of the book. Thus, she's also credited on the cover.

Foolish Assumptions

In writing this book, I'm making some basic assumptions about you. I'm assuming that:

- You have fibromyalgia, think that you have it, or have a friend or family member with FMS, and you want information in order to be able to help.
- You want information on pain relief and remedies.
- You're curious about alternative remedies and treatments.

How This Book Is Organized

Fibromyalgia For Dummies is organized into seven convenient parts, starting with what fibromyalgia is and moving to who's most likely to have it, and zeroing in on the many ways to deal with the pain, fatigue, and other common symptoms fibromyalgia sufferers share. Here's how it breaks down.

Part 1: Fibromyalgia Is the Real Deal: What It Is and Is Not

In the first four chapters, I cover the realities of fibromyalgia. I offer a self-test, in case you need help in determining whether you may have FMS. The symptoms of fibromyalgia are important to understand, and I cover them in detail in Chapter 2. I also talk about possible causes of fibromyalgia in Chapter 3. Nobody knows exactly what causes FMS, but there are some intriguing theories about the perpetrators of this medical problem. Chapter 4 covers pain and its purpose, including good pain/bad pain. Most fibromyalgia pain is "bad pain," so don't imagine that I think otherwise because I don't! However, you do need to manage FMS pain, rather than having that pain manage you.

Part II: Finding Out If You Have Fibromyalgia

To know whether you may have FMS, consider patterns among people already diagnosed. You can still have FMS if you don't fit neatly into one or more of these categories, but it's less likely. This information is covered in Chapter 5. Then, moving to Chapter 6, I describe medical problems often confused with fibromyalgia, such as chronic fatigue syndrome, myofascial pain syndrome, arthritis, and thyroid disease. Some people have more than one of these medical problems — hopefully, you won't have "all the above." Next, Chapters 7 and 8 walk you through working with your primary care doctor, and, if needed, finding a new physician.

Part III: Getting to Wellness: How Fibromyalgia Is Treated

Here's where I talk about what to *do* about your fibromyalgia. I cover over-the-counter medications, such as aspirin, guaifenesin, and dextromethorphan, in Chapter 9. And I describe the gamut of prescribed remedies for FMS in Chapter 10. I then talk about some "hands-on" therapy that can help you, such as icing or heating the painful spots or applying direct massage to your hurting areas, in Chapter 11.

In Chapter 12, I cover alternative remedies and treatments that can help you feel better, such as herbs, supplements, botox treatments (not just for facial wrinkles anymore!), acupuncture, aromatherapy, and other complementary medicine choices, as well as some treatments that you really should steer clear of.

Part IV: Lifestyle Changes: What You Can Do on Your Own

There are some good non-medical lifestyle changes that you can make to ease your pain. In Chapters 13 and 14, I cover stress control using relaxation therapy, hypnotherapy, and meditation, and I provide details on how to get a good night's sleep. In Chapter 15, I include important information on exercising, losing weight, and making dietary changes that may help considerably. In Chapter 16, I cover dealing with the emotional fallout of FMS, and, if you need a therapist, I offer advice on finding a good one.

Part V: Living and Working with Fibromyalgia

You can't switch FMS off and on (if you could, it'd always be off!), and consequently, the illness affects you both at work and at home. In Chapters 17 and

18, I discuss how to help your family, friends, coworkers, and your boss to help you. Sometimes, work may become impossible, and you may need to apply for a disability — an important subject I also cover. I offer Chapter 19 for those who don't have FMS themselves but have a friend or family member who's hurting — and whom they want to help. I also include a chapter on children with fibromyalgia, Chapter 20, in case your child, or the child of someone you know, suffers from FMS.

Part VI: The Part of Tens

This part presents helpful information in lists of ten items each. You can read about ten ways to explain fibromyalgia to your family, friends, and others. Another list offers ten must-do actions when you have FMS. I also have ten ways to beat brain malaise (*fibro fog*). Last, I debunk ten myths about FMS.

Part VII: Appendixes

In this part, I provide a glossary of commonly used terms related to fibromyalgia. I also offer an appendix of over-the-counter (OTC) drugs and prescribed medications useful to patients with FMS with the brand and chemical name of the drug, common starting dosage, symptoms it combats, and side effects.

Another appendix is an Internet resource guide of interesting Web pages where you'll find resources and articles to read as well as support groups to contact online. And, in case you're not a "Nethead," I offer an appendix of helpful organizations to contact through the mail. I also provide a list of publications devoted to fibromyalgia.

Icons Used in This Book

To help you remember the important points of each chapter, this book marks certain paragraphs with the following helpful icons:

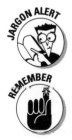

This icon marks paragraphs that define medical terms that may be unfamiliar to you.

This icon denotes critical information that you really need to take away with you. Be sure to read it.

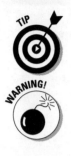

When you see this icon, you find a helpful hint for coping with fibromyalgia that may save you time or money. Or maybe both!

The Warning icon cautions you against something that's potentially harmful. Be sure to read and heed these icons.

Where to Go from Here

After you've read this book and started using my suggestions for wellness, I hope that you'll experience the improvement that many others have felt. I particularly would like you to maintain your personal commitment to managing your own health. I also hope that you'll be well armored against attacks from people out there who still (and wrongly!) think that fibromyalgia is fake. Fibromyalgia is a real medical problem; it's not something that's "in your head." But it's also a real medical problem that you can successfully combat.

Part I

Fibromyalgia Is the Real Deal: What It Is and Is Not

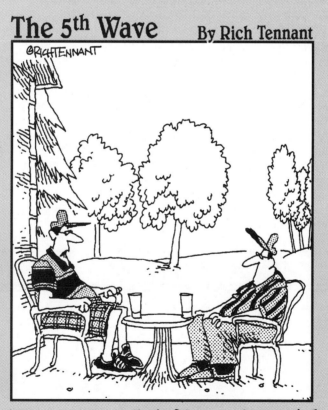

The 5th Wave   By Rich Tennant

"The doctors call it fibromyalgia, but I call it 'Military Disease' because it comes with a lot of fatigue."

In this part . . .

Fibromyalgia is the real deal — no matter what you may have heard from other people who act like they know what they're talking about. Fibromyalgia isn't "just in your head" — actually fibromyalgia pain is usually spread throughout the entire body!

In Part I, I describe the key aspects of fibromyalgia that you need to know such as what fibromyalgia is and what the symptoms are. I include a fibromyalgia self-test that you can take. I also discuss intriguing theories on why you and others may have developed fibromyalgia. I cover car crashes, infections, autoimmune systems run amuck, and other theories. Pain is the major element of fibromyalgia, and I devote an entire chapter to this topic (not at all painful to read), which may give you some good insight into what's going on with your aching body.

Chapter 1

Yes, Fibromyalgia Is Real

• •

• •

Knowing that fibromyalgia syndrome (FMS) is a real medical problem that needs to be dealt with is an important first step toward mastering your fibromyalgia — and moving toward that place where you can start to feel like you're making progress. Sure, you can try to ignore the problem. But mostly, it won't let you.

Fibromyalgia has many aspects to it to consider. In this chapter, I spell out all the major issues for you and refer you to chapters later in this book where I discuss how fibromyalgia affects you individually and what treatments and medications may work best for you.

Dumping Your Doubts about the Validity of FMS

Many people spend months or even years questioning their own bodily symptoms that stem from fibromyalgia, sometimes wondering if maybe they're imagining how bad the symptoms are. After all, if you feel terrible one day and then a lot less terrible the next day, you may start to think that maybe you were exaggerating the terrible-ness of the previous day.

The thing is, most people can't remember pain well. They can remember that they *had* pain, but they can't remember what it actually felt like. (Having a sort of pain amnesia is good!) As a result, people experiencing the ups and downs of pain and the other symptoms that accompany fibromyalgia will worry sometimes that perhaps the problem isn't that big of a deal and could even be "all in their heads." Consequently, they may try to ignore the problem, and hope that it'll go far, far away — preferably today.

But if you have fibromyalgia (and I recommend that you take my self-test at the end of this chapter to see whether you could be a possible candidate), simply ignoring the problem doesn't work. The sooner that you can acknowledge that fibromyalgia's a real problem and one that's moved into your body to stay, the sooner you can work toward reclaiming your life.

You can gain enormous control over the symptoms that stem from your fibromyalgia, but only rarely can you eradicate them altogether. Most people have plenty of room for improvement, however.

Examining the Symptoms, Causes, and Pain Problems Associated with FMS

Fibromyalgia isn't a "one size fits all" kind of medical problem, but I can make some descriptive generalizations about it regarding symptoms, causes, and pain.

Sizing up the symptoms

Many people with fibromyalgia report that the following statements are true about their fibromyalgia symptoms. In fact, most people with fibromyalgia say that they have at least several, if not all, of these following symptoms (which I cover in much more detail in Chapter 2):

- Flu-like pain that can be severe
- A constant feeling of exhaustion
- Specific tender points that hurt
- Overall body aches
- Depression
- Muscle stiffness and pain

- Insomnia or other sleep disorders
- Extreme fatigue
- Mental malaise and confusion, often referred to as *fibro fog*

Many people with FMS have other pain-based medical problems as well, which I also cover in more depth in Chapter 2. Some examples of the array of medical conditions that people with fibromyalgia may experience, on top of the fibromyalgia that they already have (as if the FMS isn't enough) include

- Irritable bowel syndrome
- Interstitial cystitis
- Arthritis
- Headaches
- Chronic fatigue syndrome

Considering causes

No one knows for sure what causes fibromyalgia, but physicians and other experts have come up with many fascinating theories to explain what might induce the onset of FMS. The cause could be hormones or an autoimmune problem or biochemicals gone awry, or it may be related to a previous trauma, such as an injury that you incurred in a car crash or in another serious accident.

The cause could also be a combination of different factors coming together at just the right time (or actually, the wrong time when you think about it) for you to develop FMS. For example, maybe you got the flu, and then you were involved in a serious car crash. Or some other awful combination may have occurred.

As researchers (like me) continue to study this medical problem, they continue to get closer to the truth. Speculating about causes can be fascinating, and Chapter 3 offers some common theories for what causes fibromyalgia.

Pondering pain

Thinking about pain is certainly no fun, and yet pain is part of what makes us alive and human. But when pain runs rampant in our bodies, extracting particular pain in certain parts of it, it becomes a problem, and fibromyalgia pain can be very intense. I talk about the purpose of pain and how and why it needs to be managed in Chapter 4. It may sound like a chapter to avoid, but wait! You should really read it because this chapter includes some important and useful ideas.

And by the way, I'm not just *saying* that I believe that the pain and symptoms of fibromyalgia are real because I'm a sympathetic, nice, or polite person. I think that I *am* those things, too, but even more important, I'm also a physician who's a clinical researcher, and I've proven in my studies on the pain of people with fibromyalgia that their pain (and yours) is real.

My studies, as well as the studies that have been done by other researchers, have shown that the pain sensations experienced by people with fibromyalgia (especially women) are actually more intense, and the pain lasts longer than does the pain of people who don't have fibromyalgia. Read Chapter 4 for further information on the ins and outs of fibromyalgia pain.

Considering Who Gets FMS

Just about anyone of any age can develop fibromyalgia, but most research so far indicates that the majority of people with FMS are of the female persuasion, partly because women suffer musculoskeletal pain more frequently than men. This is a time where a little equal opportunity of pain would be preferable (if you're a woman). But who gets fibromyalgia isn't about fairness. Instead, it's about (groan) the way things are.

Although women appear to be the primary sufferers of fibromyalgia, men have been diagnosed with FMS, too. For more info about some of the major patterns that have been identified so far among people who develop fibromyalgia, and which you may share with these kindred spirits, be sure to read Chapter 5.

What about children? Do they have fibromyalgia? Sadly, yes. If your child has FMS, he or she may have a difficult time because most physicians as well as the general public still don't know that kids can experience chronic pain from FMS. Instead, they think that the kids are faking it when they say that they're too sick to go to school. Maybe they are, but maybe not. Skip ahead to Chapter 20 for some advice on how to tell the difference.

Looking at Related Medical Problems

Sometimes, people strongly suspect (or think that they're *sure*) that they have fibromyalgia. Instead, however, they may have arthritis, Lyme disease, chronic fatigue syndrome, or a variety of other common and not-so-common medical problems. And sometimes (and maybe you can guess what's coming next), people have both fibromyalgia *and* other serious medical problems. Having fibromyalgia doesn't exempt you from getting sick with other illnesses. (Even though it seems like it should.)

With the existing array of possible medical problems and their often-overlapping symptoms, even doctors can become confused sometimes about which is which when they're working on a diagnosis. A good doctor is up to this task, of course, as long as you don't expect instant results on your first visit.

For example, suppose that one of your primary symptoms is extreme fatigue, possibly to the point of total exhaustion — even though you haven't been doing anything more strenuous than clicking the TV controller to change channels. This action may use up one calorie or less, but you feel like you've climbed Mount Everest. Maybe your problem is fibromyalgia, but maybe not.

Extreme tiredness is one of the possible symptoms of hypothyroidism, chronic fatigue syndrome, Lyme disease, arthritis, and, oh yes, fibromyalgia, too. No wonder sorting it all out can be so hard sometimes! To find out more about illnesses often confused with FMS, and how doctors sort them out, read Chapter 6.

Finding a Doctor Who's a "True Believer" in Fibromyalgia

Although I believe that most intelligent and well-educated physicians are at least *aware* of the existence of fibromyalgia and its basic symptoms, and they also know that it's a valid problem that needs to be treated, I also know that a few doctors out there still haven't gotten the word yet. If your doctor isn't helping you with your FMS symptoms, you need to help him understand it. (Maybe asking him if he's read this book would be a good start.)

A good doctor will consider your symptoms as valid, take a complete medical history, and perform a physical examination. Read Chapters 7 and 8 for more details.

Sometimes, no matter what you do, a particular physician isn't working out for you. Maybe the two of you have a personality conflict, or maybe he thinks that you should just tough out your fibromyalgia. Or maybe the problem stems from something else altogether. Whatever it is, sometimes, you just need to find a new doctor. (And I've devoted a significant part of Chapter 7 to help you find a new doc, if that's what you need to do.)

After you find a good doctor who's interested in working with you, she can formulate a plan for you to follow — one that's doable in your life. Usually, such a plan involves medications to take (over-the-counter and/or prescribed drugs and, sometimes, supplements or alternative remedies, too) as well as advice on basic lifestyle changes that you can make to improve your health. Some of these lifestyle changes may involve foods to eat or not eat, exercises to perform, and other therapies that may improve your symptoms.

Treating the Problem

When you have fibromyalgia, at least some of the time, you need to take some medications, whether they're over-the-counter drugs; prescribed medications, such as muscle relaxants or painkillers; or other medications that can help to ease your pain and your symptoms. I cover these topics thoroughly in Chapters 9 and 10. You can also often gain benefit from what I call "hands-on" therapy, including heat, ice, and other fascinating physical contact choices (such as massage or mud baths) that I cover in Chapter 11.

And don't forget about the promise of alternative remedies! People with fibromyalgia have some very intriguing choices to consider, ranging from acupuncture to biofeedback to botox. Read more details about all the different choices in Chapter 12.

Making Lifestyle Changes: Pulling Yourself into a Non-Fibro World

As you work to pull yourself farther back into the non-fibromyalgia world, you may sometimes feel like a person loaded down with 50 pounds of extra weight, trying to slog your way through the swamp. During your struggle you watch others on dry land with no heavy packs dart by you, maybe waving at you and telling you that they'll see you later on.

If you want to improve your life quality and be able to reduce your backpack of troublesome symptoms, consider the following basic ideas:

✓ **De-stress yourself.** Stress is a normal part of life, but if you have fibromyalgia on top of the usual daily stresses, or maybe with some extra stress thrown in once in awhile, you're in a bad situation. Stress can greatly worsen the chronic pain, fatigue, and other symptoms of the person with fibromyalgia. Be sure to read Chapter 13 for my suggestions on relaxation therapy, hypnosis, meditation, T'ai Chi, and other methods to "de-stress" yourself. They work!

✔ **Improve your sleep to decrease your pain.** Don't kid yourself. Five or even six hours of sleep each night aren't enough. So, if insufficient sleep is a problem for you, as it is for many people with fibromyalgia, face up to it. You may need medication, an alternative remedy, or another form of treatment to solve this no- or low-sleep problem that you're going through. Read Chapter 14 for some ideas on how to resolve sleep problems and help yourself feel better.

✔ **Exercise.** Unless you're an exercise-aholic, you probably don't like the idea of exercising (most people don't), and the mere thought of it may be nearly migraine inducing for some readers. But the fact is, exercise will usually help you to limber up and lose weight, making you more mobile and also helping you to feel better.

Exercise shouldn't hurt a lot, nor should it be really unpleasant and something to dread. If you hate swimming or bicycling, don't use those activities as your exercises. Maybe walking would suit you better, or maybe dancing or some other form of aerobic exercise with your partner or a friend. You can exercise in many different ways: Be creative and find the best ways for you. (I provide some FMS-friendly exercise ideas in Chapter 15.)

✔ **Pay attention to your emotions.** Stress isn't the only problem that people with fibromyalgia often face. Depression and anxiety are also very common, and they may be problems that you face. These problems are treatable and, in Chapter 16, I talk about how to know if you may have a problem, and how to identify a good therapist to help you, if you need one.

Coping with Fibromyalgia at Home and on the Job

Unfortunately, fibromyalgia doesn't end at 6 p.m. or whenever you arrive home from work, nor does it go away when you wake up in the morning, struggling to get ready for another day at work or at home. When you have FMS, it's always there on the sidelines, waiting to jump on you yet again with its aggravating symptoms.

You also need to keep in mind that other people you interact with on a daily basis (your partner, children, friends, coworkers, and other family members) are directly affected by your fibromyalgia, even if they don't have FMS themselves.

Virtually anyone you interact with on a regular basis needs to have some understanding of what you need from them, whether you tell them that you have fibromyalgia or not. (Some people tell everyone that they have "arthritis" because they think that it sounds better.)

Even as you become more aware of your symptoms and how best to resolve them, you still have to deal with the "non-fibro" world, comprised of your family members who don't have fibromyalgia, your fellow workers, and many others you interact with. You need to develop workable strategies to cope with these varying situations and come up with a winning game plan for your life. I cover these topics in Chapters 17 and 18.

Working with FMS at work

Many people with fibromyalgia continue to work full-time or part-time, despite their pain and fatigue. They struggle with what to do when their symptoms make it hard to continue to work.

Sorting out the issues

Many people worry about whether they should tell others at work about their FMS, who they should tell, what they should say, and so much more. In Chapter 17, I provide a thorough overview of these issues and how they've affected real people. I also include advice from an attorney who's an expert in getting people with FMS approved for Social Security disability.

Managing managed care mania

You may also be struggling with your insurance company on paying for seeing specialists or receiving treatments that you need to treat your FMS. Chapter 17 includes some insider advice on coping with the managed care mavens.

Handling FMS with family and friends

Even the most loving family members and friends usually don't really "get" fibromyalgia if they don't have it themselves. And even if they do have FMS, too, their symptoms may be very different from what you experience, and the intensity of them may be better or worse than the way your symptoms grab hold of you.

As nice as it would be if this were true, the reality is that fibromyalgia isn't a quickie one-time explanation. For people to understand what your problem is, especially the people with whom you share your home and your life, helping them get a clue about what you're going through and what you need takes a lot of work.

You have to be candid, and you also need to know how to respond to the dumb things that people often say to people who have fibromyalgia. Read Chapter 18 for more information on how (and also how not) to explain fibromyalgia to your children of all ages, your partner, and other family members and friends, so that they can better understand what's really going on here.

Don't miss the information that I provide on sex and fibromyalgia for readers who are sensing that their partners are maybe feeling a teensy bit deprived in this area of life. (Thinking about sex when you hurt is a hard thing to do, but it's not hard for your non-FMS partner to think about it. Finding common ground is a good idea.)

Sorting it out when you don't have fibromyalgia

Maybe you don't have fibromyalgia, but you live with someone who does, and you really want to understand the problem and to help as much as possible. But where do you begin? Not to worry, I've provided a chapter just for you — Chapter 19.

This chapter describes techniques to assist you in helping your friend or loved one deal with FMS, and it also tells you some things you should not do or say because they drive most people with fibromyalgia wild. (People who do have fibromyalgia may enjoy reading Chapter 19, too, and sharing it with their friends and family members who don't have FMS.)

Do You Have Fibromyalgia? A Self-test

Only your physician can diagnose you with fibromyalgia and then treat you. Reading this book is a very good idea, but it still doesn't really cut it when it comes to making an actual diagnosis in your own individual case. What I can give you is a simple self-test to use to help you determine if you *may* have fibromyalgia syndrome.

Grab a scratch piece of paper and jot down your answers to the following "yes" or "no" questions. Then, read my analysis at the end of the list. If you think that you may be a possible candidate for fibromyalgia, make an appointment with your physician and find out for sure.

1. **Do you have a lot of pain in certain specific areas of your body? If so, do the areas lack any obvious damage (such as bruising or swelling)?**

2. Is your body pain sometimes severe?

3. Do you have trouble sleeping on three or more nights per week?

4. Do you feel exhausted about half the time or more?

5. Do people often ask you if you're sick?

6. Do you turn down social invitations rather than risk having to go out feeling achy and tired?

7. Do you find yourself wondering whether your aches and pains will ever go away or if you'll feel like this forever?

8. Are you always losing things and forgetting things? Do you have so much mental confusion that you sometimes wonder if it could be an early onset of Alzheimer's disease?

9. Are you having trouble finding a pattern to your pain — some days it's bad and some days it's not?

10. Have you started to feel really "down" about the pain and fatigue that you've been experiencing? Are you wondering if depression could be the problem?

If you answered "yes" to as many as three or more of these questions, you may have fibromyalgia, although every person's case is different. That's why even if you only answered "yes" to one or two of my questions, but you think that you may have fibromyalgia, a consultation with your physician is a good idea.

Now, here's some explanation of what may be happening to you, depending on your answers to Questions 1 through 10. Keep in mind, though, that only your doctor can actually diagnose you with fibromyalgia.

✔ **Question 1:** If you're experiencing pain in specific parts of your body, but you're not seeing any bruises or any apparent evidence of damage (and neither is your doctor), these painful areas may be the "tender points" that are characteristic of fibromyalgia. Read Chapter 8 for more information on tender points.

✔ **Question 2:** If you said that your pain is sometimes very severe, this is another indicator that you may have fibromyalgia. Be sure to consult with a physician to find out.

✔ **Question 3:** If you have trouble sleeping three or more nights per week, you have a serious problem. The problem may or may not be connected with fibromyalgia (although nearly everyone with FMS has sleep problems), but you need to resolve the serious sleep deficit you're building up. If you're a walking zombie because you're not getting enough sleep, you can't perform well at work or home, nor will you be a happy person.

Also, if you're prone to developing fibromyalgia, this continuing bad pattern of a lack of sleep every night will make your other symptoms, such as your pain and fatigue, much worse.

✔ **Question 4:** Severe fatigue is a chronic problem among nearly everyone who has fibromyalgia. Often, it's linked to a lack of sleep. But it may also be an element of FMS as a medical problem. You may also have chronic fatigue syndrome, and your doctor will need to help you sort it out.

✔ **Question 5:** If you agreed that those you care about, or maybe even strangers around you, are asking you if you're ill, something about you probably doesn't look right. You may be displaying your chronic pain on your face without even knowing it.

On the other hand, other people tell individuals with fibromyalgia that they look "fine" and "great," and the pain and symptoms aren't reflected in the face or body language of the fibro sufferer. If this has happened to you, you're definitely not alone.

✔ **Question 6:** If you're turning down a lot of invitations that you would have accepted in the past, you really need to have a serious talk with yourself to find out the reason why. Is it because of pain and fatigue? Or could you be having a problem with depression — a very common problem and highly treatable for people with and without fibromyalgia?

✔ **Question 7:** When your pain is constant and chronic, asking yourself if it's ever going to end is only natural. But what you do need to do is consult with a physician. You may have fibromyalgia, or you may have another problem altogether.

✔ **Question 8:** If you constantly lose things or forget things, you may have the mental confusion that stems from fibromyalgia. You may also have attention deficit disorder. You may also be trying to do too many things at once, and you need to take some items off your plate.

How do you know which it is? You make a stab at analyzing what you're forgetting and when. If you can't even begin to do that, and you also are experiencing chronic pain, fatigue, and sleep problems, you may have fibromyalgia. See your doctor to find out for sure.

✔ **Question 9:** If your pain is severe on some days and then far less of a problem on other days, and you think there doesn't seem to be any sort of pattern to it at all, you may be seeing the chronic ups and downs of fibromyalgia.

Widespread pain that can appear in one part of your body one day and migrate elsewhere on another day is common, as are days when you feel really bad, bad, and only mildly bad.

✔ **Question 10:** If you've been feeling pretty melancholy and maybe sort of overwhelmed by all your many aches and pains, you may have depression. Many people with fibromyalgia have both depression and FMS.

But before rushing off to the nearest psychiatrist to ask for Zoloft or the latest antidepressant approved last week by the Food and Drug Administration (FDA), as a first step, consider talking to your regular doctor or to a rheumatologist. Why? Your primary problem may actually be fibromyalgia, and if your medical problem is treated and then your symptoms subsequently improve, so may your sad mood. Many doctors prescribe antidepressant medications to treat pain *and* FMS. Get more details on this in Chapter 10.

This test is just a starting point. If you're really concerned that you may have FMS and/or another chronic illness, don't hesitate to make an appointment with your doctor.

Chapter 2

Recognizing Key Symptoms of Fibromyalgia

*F*or Sandy, the horrible pain is what bothers her the most about her fibromyalgia. Sure, she has some other symptoms that bother her as well, such as fatigue and chronic muscle stiffness, especially in the morning. But really only the severe pain counts, in her mind.

For Lisa, the pain is also terrible, but she thinks that if she just weren't so horribly tired *all* the time, then maybe the pain drugs that she takes would enable her to actually accomplish something — anything. As it is, she feels like she's trapped in quicksand. She's not going down and under because she's not thrashing about. But she's not actually moving anywhere, either.

Andy, another person with fibromyalgia, says that he feels overwhelmed by *everything*. The pain. The constant tiredness. The confusion. The frequent headaches. Andy wants it all to go away — preferably right now.

In this chapter, I cover the key symptoms of fibromyalgia, including — first and foremost — the pain and stiffness that nearly everyone complains about. I also cover the extreme fatigue that causes constant problems for most people with fibromyalgia syndrome (FMS). In addition, I include information on what some people with fibromyalgia call *brain fog* or *fibro fog* that's really a sort of temporary mental confusion resulting in difficulty concentrating.

I also cover the syndromes and diseases that are most commonly associated with fibromyalgia, such as *irritable bowel syndrome* (IBS), *interstitial cystitis*

(IC), chronic headaches, chronic heartburn, depression, and arthritic conditions. You may be interested to discover that some of the treatments for these individual ailments are similar to (or exactly the same as) the treatments that are recommended for fibromyalgia.

Describing Where It Hurts: Everywhere!

Most people with fibromyalgia say that the widespread pain drives them the most crazy. Sure, they don't like the fatigue or muscle aches, nor do they enjoy the fibro fog. These symptoms are common for many people with FMS. But they may seem minor league compared to the hurting-all-over pain, which can sometimes escalate from mild or moderate to severe pain.

Eva has had FMS for years, so she has an up-close and personal relationship with the illness. Eva says that to understand how FMS feels, imagine that a gigantic truck just ran over you — and then backed up and ran you over again.

Feeling aches and body pains of your FMS — but unable to show proof

You probably find it hard to explain to people *where* you hurt. You can get some pretty strange looks when you say that you hurt *everywhere*. Not just in your back or in your legs or your neck or in other sites of your body. All those places may hurt, and maybe some other places, too. Nor do you have any visible damage that you can point to. No broken bones, no gushing wounds, not even one bruise that you can single out to show someone, "*Here*, this is where it hurts me the most. Look at this."

Laboratory tests can't diagnose fibromyalgia — at least, not yet. Tests can only tell you that you don't have other medical problems. You shouldn't, therefore, be alarmed or surprised if doctors can't find anything except some *tender points,* where you wince more when pressure is applied there than when they touch you elsewhere. (Read more about the tender points of fibromyalgia in Chapter 8.)

So you've got no hard evidence that you can present for your pain. And yet, you continue to hurt and hurt and hurt and hurt.

As an FMS sufferer, you're not alone in regard to a lack of specific laboratory findings. People with migraine headaches, tension headaches, and back pain have chronic recurrent pain. Many chronic pain conditions lack overt physical findings. Most important, you need to remember that you don't have to prove that you hurt. You know that you have pain, and that's good enough. Instead, you need to focus on finding a knowledgeable doctor who can diagnose your illness. In order to diagnose you with FMS, for example, he or she needs to consider several different conditions that may mimic this chronic pain syndrome. Just to reassure you, a doctor who takes a good history and performs a careful physical examination can diagnose most FMS sufferers. (See Chapter 7 for advice on finding a good fibromyalgia doctor.)

Suffering from muscle stiffness (especially in the morning)

Many people with fibromyalgia say that the severe muscle stiffness and achiness is at its worst in the morning. You may wake up to a new day and feel like you've participated in a major marathon — or maybe gremlins were beating on you all night long. The stiffness may diminish as you move about, but it usually doesn't go away completely. People with arthritis also often experience muscle stiffness, and maybe in the past, doctors told you that your problem was arthritis.

You may have both arthritis *and* fibromyalgia. Having fibromyalgia doesn't (unfortunately) exempt you from other medical problems. If you do suffer from chronic stiffness, read Chapter 15, which includes some good, easy stretching exercises to help you with this problem.

Tammy, whose fibromyalgia was diagnosed several years ago, feels that one of the hardest parts for her is dealing with the severe morning stiffness that she suffers from. In fact, when she gets up in the morning or rises after sitting for a long period, she has such a hard time that her husband calls her contortions to get up her "rigor mortis walk" because her movements look so torturous and stiff. (Tammy says that she doesn't mind his teasing because he's supportive and understanding of the problems that she faces with fibromyalgia.)

Pinpointing the source of your pain: You can't

When you try to analyze exactly where all this pain is coming from — the master source — you just can't figure it out. Nor can you deduce *why* you're experiencing it. Your doctor may often be very puzzled by these questions, too.

Some experts believe that extreme exercise may induce FMS. But you probably *haven't* been exercising like crazy because you feel too bad to exercise a lot (or at all). You probably haven't just fallen or had some other accident or injury, either, although some researchers believe that a severe injury or car crash actually can trigger fibromyalgia in some people. (Read more about possible causes of fibromyalgia in Chapter 3.)

Chronically feeling your pain

Another key aspect of fibromyalgia is that the pain is *chronic,* which means that (so sorry) it's sticking around. Sometimes, it's better; sometimes, it's worse. But it always seems to be *there,* sort of waiting to ambush you when you let your guard down. Time to go out to the big annual dinner at work! All of a sudden, the pain escalates to newer, excruciatingly high levels. Stress often aggravates fibromyalgia, and as a result, the pain can flare up at the worst of times.

Are you suffering from *oligoanalgesia*? This word refers to the undertreatment, ineffectual treatment, or total *non*treatment of pain — a problem that many people with fibromyalgia can relate to. Yet both nontreatment and inadequate treatment of pain can seriously weaken your immune system and can also impair your quality of life. Read Chapter 4 for more information on pain and its role in your life. (Everyone who reads this book definitely needs to read that chapter.)

Migrating pain: The worst pain may move from place to place

Another truly maddening aspect of FMS is that the worst pain can be in your lower back today, your neck tomorrow, and maybe your upper back the next day. Or maybe your whole spinal column is doing okay right now, but you're having a serious problem with pain from irritable bowel syndrome or headaches — both common conditions for people with fibromyalgia. Or perhaps you suffer from a combination of medical problems, which happens frequently.

Pam says that her fibromyalgia feels like a kind of radiating pain that pops up like a poltergeist in new places all the time. She never knows when or where it'll hit her next.

Fibromyalgia isn't the only chronic syndrome. The fact is, many medical problems that people suffer from today are chronic ones. High blood pressure is a chronic problem for many people; diabetes is another. Many people also suffer from chronic back pain. You're not alone is experiencing a chronic disease.

Feeling Extremely Fatigued

Darla says that sometimes she gives the orders to her feet to go, but they just don't move, and this is especially true when she first gets up in the morning.

As if the other symptoms weren't enough. . .

Some people with FMS suffer from an array of other symptoms beyond pain, fatigue, sleep difficulties, brain fog, and so forth. Here are some of these annoying, but more unusual, symptoms:

- **Restless legs:** People with this symptom get a feeling of excitability and irritability in the legs (sometimes at night when lying still in bed) that makes them feel compelled to move about or shake their legs.

- **Paresthesia:** Also known as "pins and needles," this symptom primarily affects the legs, hands, or feet of fibromyalgia sufferers.

- **Tinnitus:** A ringing in the ears is a problem that some people with fibromyalgia experience.

Of course, these symptoms may be caused by other medical problems, so if you have them, be sure to let your doctor know.

This extreme fatigue is quite common among people with fibromyalgia. Yet, despite such profound fatigue, few patients find themselves able to get a satisfactory night's sleep. Although the pain is still the worst part for most people with FMS, the bone-numbing exhaustion is also terribly distressing for many people who say that this kind of fatigue goes well beyond simple tiredness.

Falling down exhausted

If you actually *were* exercising vigorously, you could understand this pain and exhaustion. But if you've been in "couch potato" mode and have been sitting or lying down all day (because it hurt you to move even from one position to another), you can feel really frustrated when doing nothing seems to take all the energy you've got.

Your frustration may increase when you hear that you should be sure to exercise. What? When you can barely drag your body out of bed or from the chair? Is your doctor totally nuts? (Well, no, actually exercise *is* good advice. I tell you why in Chapter 15, and I recommend some basic exercises to try, too. Be sure to read it!)

Considering whether you have chronic fatigue syndrome

Some people who haven't been diagnosed with FMS yet are so extremely tired that they wonder if they really may have *chronic fatigue syndrome* (CFS), a medical problem characterized by extreme exhaustion. (Read Chapter 6 for more information on CFS.) In general, if pain is the prevailing symptom and other symptoms of fibromyalgia are also present, you more than likely have fibromyalgia rather than chronic fatigue syndrome.

But, of course, a physician must make this determination. Don't try to diagnose yourself. And by the way, it's also possible to have *both* CFS and fibromyalgia. Hopefully, though, that's not the case with you.

Facing Fibro Fog: Mental Malaise

Many people say that the mental confusion and forgetfulness, particularly attention and concentration difficulties, are what really bothers them. People with fibromyalgia are bookkeepers, attorneys, doctors, salespeople, teachers, and so on. All these careers require mental alertness. But let's face it, you can have the easiest job in the world, and it still requires more mental acuity than you can muster up in the middle of a fibro fog attack — even if you're a certified genius.

If you can hang on to your sense of humor, it can help you relax — at least a little bit. In fact, you really *need* a sense of humor with fibromyalgia. Linda was diagnosed with fibromyalgia several years ago, and she says a sense of humor helps a lot. She recalls pouring cereal on a dinner plate, followed by the milk, and then realizing: Oops! That wasn't a bowl she was filling up. She finds that laughing at her absent-mindedness from the brain fog helps a lot.

Feeling "out of it"

You may feel like one of those walking zombies that you see in late-night movies. Feeling like you're a sleepwalker through life, rather than an active participant in it, can be hard.

Avoid blaming yourself or labeling yourself as a stupid, crazy, or bad person. Do the best you can. That's all that anyone (including yourself) should expect from you. Still, dealing with it can be hard. Judy says that her fibromyalgia developed about a year after she was treated for Graves' Disease, a form of *hyperthyroidism* (overactive thyroid gland). She says that she wants her brain back the way it was — and right now. She's tired of forgetting words, ideas, and people.

Being frequently inattentive

You probably have a hard time paying attention to what's going on around you when you're saddled with the mental malaise that's so characteristic of fibromyalgia. Sure, you'd love to be an effective listener and be actively involved, but it's just not possible now. It's not that you don't care about your friends or that you don't love your family members. You do. You just can't help being so inattentive on so many occasions.

It's sort of like being temporarily bogged down in some major mud. Normally, you stride along, accomplishing your daily tasks at a regular pace. But when you're hit with fibro fog, it's like slogging through a deep mental mire. It's also much harder to pay attention when you're so distracted by this mental slow-down. (Be sure to read Chapter 18 on how to help your friends, family members, and other people you care about understand fibromyalgia and what's going on with you.)

Wondering about attention deficit disorder

You may wonder whether your real problem could actually be *attention deficit disorder* (ADD), a syndrome characterized by disorganization, distractibility, and forgetfulness. Although most people first think of children when they think of attention deficit disorder, adults can have ADD, too. But if your primary problem is chronic pain "all over" that doctors can't attribute to anything other than fibromyalgia, FMS is likely to be what you have. (Of course, as with other conditions, you can have both fibromyalgia and ADD.)

Coping with temporary confusion

Coping with your temporary mental confusion can be very difficult. After all, how can you solve a problem when you're unable to pay attention to the task at hand or concentrate on it? It's also true that stress can trigger or worsen your distractibility. The trick is to find remedies when you're not confused that will work (or at least, help) during those times when you *are* confused.

You may want to try some of the same types of tricks that help people with ADD to cope with confusion, such as creating simple lists, always keeping your car keys in the same place, and quickly checking yourself in the mirror before you leave the house. (Yes, your clothes are right side out, and they're on you, and your hair is combed. Or they aren't, so you fix them.)

Weathering Your Reactions to Weather

Many people with fibromyalgia feel that they're very *weather-sensitive*. When a cold or warm front is coming on, before they ever hear it on the radio or see a TV report about the impending storm, they already feel the pain intensifying in their bodies. Major temperature changes may also cause your fibromyalgia symptoms to flare up. Cold and wet weather seems to bother weather-sensitive fibromyalgia sufferers the most.

Some people actually study this phenomenon of weather changes and their impact: It's called *biometeorology*, or the study of how the weather (changes in air pressure, precipitation, temperature, wind, and so forth) can affect people's bodies.

People who have increased fibromyalgia pain with weather changes have reported to researchers that the worst months for them are November and December, and the best month is July. However, you shouldn't count on July as being a no-pain month, nor should you basically go into hibernation at the end of October. In fact, you may actually notice no differences in those months at all because individual reactions to weather vary.

Some anecdotal reports indicate that women may be more weather-sensitive than men are. Of course, how you feel really depends on your individual circumstances, the type of climate that you live in, and other factors. In general, most people with fibromyalgia do better in milder climates. However, experts say that if you're a weather-sensitive person with fibromyalgia, relocating to a warm, dry climate won't automatically make you feel *completely* well. You may feel better, but don't assume that moving to Arizona will mean a cure for you. It usually won't.

Dealing with Common Sleep Disorders

Difficulty with sleeping is an extremely common problem for people with fibromyalgia. In fact, if you don't have this problem, you're unusual — and maybe you don't have fibromyalgia at all. (On the other hand, maybe whatever you're doing to combat your sleep disorder is working well, and that's good.)

Fibromyalgia pain often serves as the cause for insomnia and other sleep disorders. In a vicious cycle, the lack of sleep usually makes you feel worse, which in turn, makes it even harder for you to sleep the next night. You can build up a serious sleep deficit. Solutions, however, are available. If you suffer from chronic insomnia or other sleep problems, be sure to read Chapter 14 to find out more about how to improve your sleep cycles.

Experiencing Related Medical Problems

Many people with fibromyalgia also suffer from a variety of other pain-based medical problems that affect the digestive system, the joints, the nerves, and the mind such as

✔ Irritable bowel syndrome (IBS)

✔ Interstitial cystitis (IC)

✔ Osteoarthritis

✔ Rheumatoid arthritis

Experts don't know why these types of painful problems seem to go together, but they have plenty of theories to explain it. One theory is that the system that controls pain — whether it's a neurochemical, hormone, or something else — has gone awry. As a result, the afflicted person can suffer from a variety of painful conditions. (Read more about possible causes of fibromyalgia in Chapter 3.)

Dealing with irritable bowel syndrome

Having the pain, achiness, and mental confusion that can accompany fibromyalgia is bad enough. But many people also suffer from *irritable bowel syndrome* (IBS), a colonic condition that, very simply put, causes the person to alternate between having constipation and diarrhea. (Another name for IBS is *spastic colon.*)

You either can't go at all, or you're constantly running for the bathroom. Which condition is worse is up to you. (Probably whatever you're suffering from right now.) Some people with IBS have *only* chronic constipation or *only* chronic diarrhea, though, and don't switch back and forth between these two extreme conditions.

Studies indicate that about 15 percent of adults in the U.S. have symptoms that indicate that they have IBS, and the disease is apparently about 3 times more prominent among women. (Although men may have IBS a lot and report it much less — researchers aren't really sure.)

As with fibromyalgia, experts disagree on what actually causes IBS, although most of them concur that stress makes it worse. Most experts also agree that certain types of foods can aggravate IBS. Interestingly, some of the same foods that can cause a flare-up of fibromyalgia can also worsen IBS, such as citrus fruits, chocolate, and alcohol, to name the leading culprits.

Diagnosing

Your primary care doctor can usually diagnose and treat IBS, although he or she may want to refer you to a *gastroenterologist*, a specialist in digestive diseases. Based on your physical examination and a review of your medical history, the gastroenterologist may decide to do a *colonoscopy*, which is an internal view of your colon while you're under mild sedation. This procedure is especially likely to be done if you're over age 50 or if you're at risk for developing colorectal cancer. When the doctor examines your colon from the inside with a special scope, he or she will be able to see any indications of disease.

Treating IBS

How is IBS treated? The doctor will almost always urge you to increase your intake of vegetables and cut back (or eliminate) alcohol and chocolate. Medication can help and, thankfully, sometimes the same sort of drugs that help a person with fibromyalgia can also alleviate some of the symptoms of IBS. For example, a very low dose of an antidepressant such as *Elavil* (generic name: amitriptyline), may help ease IBS symptoms as well as FMS symptoms.

Coping with interstitial cystitis

Some people with fibromyalgia suffer from a painful bladder condition called *interstitial cystitis* (IC). This chronic and sometimes severe condition basically makes the person who has it feel like she (or he, although most sufferers are female) has to urgently urinate constantly. She feels this way even after she just went to the bathroom, and she *knows* she just urinated. The condition may feel like a bladder infection, but no bacteria can be found when the urine is tested.

Often, the bladder aches painfully, sort of like having one or more canker sores on your bladder's sensitive tissue. Many people with IC have been treated with repeated courses of antibiotics because doctors assumed that they must have had bladder infections, despite a negative urinalysis, because they were in such pain. Yet unnecessary antibiotics can aggravate the painful bladder even further.

Experts don't know what causes IC, but it may be a reaction to a previous infection, or it could have an autoimmune basis — meaning that the immune system turns on itself and attacks its own tissue.

Diagnosing IC

Because IC is considered a rare disease, most primary care physicians find it difficult to diagnose. Generally, *urologists*, physicians specializing in diseases of the urinary tract, will diagnose IC.

In the case of most people who think they may have (or do have) a bladder infection, many doctors recommend drinking copious quantities of cranberry juice to help stave it off and maybe even stop an early infection cold in its tracks. But don't do this if you have IC! Your bladder is unusually sensitive already, and the high acidity of cranberry juice will only accelerate the spasms and the pain. Instead, ask your doctor for another remedy. And be sure to drink plenty of plain old water.

Treating IC

Chronic cases of IC can be treated with medications that are instilled directly into the bladder through a catheter. Patients can also take certain oral medicines that may calm down the bladder spasms.

As with IBS, some of the same medications that help other symptoms of fibromyalgia may help the person with IC. For example, Elavil may help with the pain from IC. In addition, antihistamines are often used to treat IC.

Doctors also often recommend dietary changes. As with IBS and other conditions commonly experienced by patients with FMS, doctors often advise IC patients to avoid citrus fruits, chocolate, and alcohol.

In his book, *The Interstitial Cystitis Survival Guide* (New Harbinger Publications, 2000), author Robert M. Moldwin, MD acknowledges that many people with interstitial cystitis also suffer from fibromyalgia. Dr. Moldwin offers many helpful hints on medications and therapies that can help people who suffer from IC. He's also one of the few males who's been diagnosed with IC.

Aching with arthritis

Joint inflammations can be very painful, worsening the already-existing problem of fibromyalgia. Sometimes people who have fibromyalgia only are diagnosed with arthritis instead. They may be treated with anti-inflammatory drugs and other medications that often work well for people with arthritis and yet do little or nothing for people who have FMS.

Diagnosing arthritis

Arthritis isn't a tough call for most doctors to diagnose, although some rarer forms, such as lupus, can be tricky. *Rheumatologists* specialize in treating arthritis and other diseases of the joints, bones, and muscles.

In general, the diagnosis of arthritis is based on the doctor's findings during the physical examination combined with the results from x-ray and laboratory tests that the doctor ordered. (Read Chapter 8 for more information on the physical examination and diagnosis of fibromyalgia.)

Doctors can check for *rheumatoid arthritis*, a severe form of arthritis in which the body's immune system turns upon and attacks itself. This disease may be detected with a special blood test that can identify a factor also found in several other inflammatory conditions. If this factor is not found, you may not have any of these conditions.

Patients with rheumatoid arthritis are at risk for developing joint erosions, joint destruction, and severe physical deformities and disability in addition to the inflammation of other organs. They may be treated with anti-inflammatory medications and ice. They are often also treated with one or more disease-modifying drugs that are specific to the treatment of rheumatoid arthritis, such as Rheumtrex (generic name: Methotexate), Enbrel (generic name: etanercept), and Remicade (generic name: inflixamab).

You may, however, have *osteoarthritis,* which is a common disease that causes the progressive deterioration of the cartilage and joints of your body. It often comes with aging, although you can be in your thirties or younger when osteoarthritis first starts to become a problem for you. Very simply, osteoarthritis causes pain and inflammation of your joints. It can often be detected in x-rays of your bones. The doctor will usually order an x-ray of the part of your body that bothers you the most, whether it's your back, neck, hand, or another part of your musculoskeletal system.

Treating arthritis

How your arthritis is treated depends on how severe it is, how long you've had it, and many other factors. Generally, arthritis is treated with over-the-counter or prescribed medications, such as anti-inflammatory drugs, as well as with heating or icing the painful area or sometimes with massage. (Flip to Chapter 11 for more information on hands-on therapies, such as icing and heating your pain problems.)

The doctor may also prescribe a muscle relaxant, if your muscles appear to be spasming around the damaged joint. Painkillers are frequently prescribed, ranging from over the counter ibuprofen to very strong narcotics. What the doctor recommends depends on the patient and the situation.

Suffering from migraines and/or tension headaches

Do you suffer from FMS as well as regular bouts with severe headaches? If so, you're certainly not alone. No one knows how many people with fibromyalgia suffer from periodic migraines or from tension headaches, but doctors do know, based upon what their patients tell them, that they happen a lot. The underlying problem could be that whatever it is in the body that controls pain has gone wrong. Or it could be that the body is overly sensitive to pain. It might even be both.

Diagnosing headaches

A *migraine* headache is a special kind of headache that can be extremely severe and is often accompanied by nausea and vomiting. The pain is usually excruciating; people often describe it as "blinding."

Some people have special experiences called *auras* before the pain of the migraine begins, ranging from seeing strange lights to smelling something that isn't there to other auras. People with migraines often complain that light and sounds bother them, and they generally want to lie down in a dark place alone and in the same position for as long as possible. (Or until their medication kicks in.)

A tension headache is another type of headache. It isn't necessarily caused by stress or tension, although it can be. *Tension headaches* stem from tightened muscles, often in the neck, and are very common. Virtually everyone has had a tension headache at some point. When tension headaches (or any type of headaches) become chronic, though, you need to see your doctor to get a handle on the *why* of this frequency and to rule out any serious underlying problems.

Virtually any type of doctor can diagnose headache problems, although *neurologists*, who are doctors who specialize in treating diseases of the nervous system, also treat chronic headache problems. If the headaches are constantly occurring and very severe, the doctor may order a *magnetic resonance imaging* (MRI) scan of your brain, a special test to rule out a brain tumor or other dangerous condition.

Treating your headache problem

If you have migraines or tension headaches that just happen for no apparent reason (much like your fibromyalgia), your doctor will probably treat you with painkilling medications. Drugs such as Elavil — as used with IBS, interstitial cystitis, and fibromyalgia — are often prescribed to keep these headaches under control or (even better) to prevent them from happening in the first place.

Generally, doctors also recommend that if you have chronic headaches, you should avoid acidic fruits, chocolate, and alcohol. (I'm not making this up. Are you starting to see a pattern here?) In addition, although caffeine may be used in some drugs to treat severe headaches, you'll generally be discouraged from heavy consumption of caffeinated beverages, such as coffee, tea, and colas.

Some research indicates that migraine headaches may be caused by a minor deficiency of magnesium, and thus in such cases, supplemental magnesium may help. Of course, before you even consider adding magnesium to your diet, you should first check with your doctor. Also realize that magnesium may stimulate your colon, so if you already have IBS and suffer from chronic diarrhea, magnesium may not be the right answer for you.

Hurting with heartburn

Many people who have fibromyalgia also suffer from chronic heartburn. They may have *gastroesophageal reflux disease* (GERD), a condition in which food comes partway *up* the food tube (esophagus) that connects to your stomach, instead of going down where it's supposed to go. This frequent backing up of food is also known as *acid reflux*.

The condition can be extremely irritating to the esophagus. Although the stomach has its own protective layer of mucous, the esophagus has no such protection. Chronic heartburn can wear down the esophagus and even create a precancerous condition.

Diagnosing GERD

Most primary care doctors can easily diagnose GERD. If a person appears to have the symptoms of chronic heartburn (belching, upset stomach, food that they taste repeatedly for a long time after they ate it, because some of it backs up [otherwise known as "repeating" on them], and so forth), the doctor may prescribe acid-blocking medications. If patients who take these medications feel better, then they probably had heartburn.

Sometimes doctors will refer patients with heartburn symptoms to gastroenterologists. The gastroenterologist may perform an *endoscopy*, a procedure in which the doctor looks into the esophagus and stomach while the patient is mildly sedated. The endoscopy shows if there's any serious problem. It can also confirm if GERD is present.

According to the book *How to Stop Heartburn: Simple Ways to Heal Heartburn and Acid Reflux*, by Anil Minocha, MD and Christine Adamec (Wiley), some strong painkillers, such as Oxycontin, Percocet, or Vicodin, can cause or worsen your GERD. So if you're finding that the painkiller or other medication that you are taking for your fibromyalgia seems to be worsening your heartburn, be sure to let your doctor know, so you can be switched to another type of medication.

Treating GERD

GERD is usually treated with one of a variety of different types of acid-blocking medications. People with GERD are also usually given dietary recommendations. Can you guess? No acidic fruit, chocolate, or alcohol — just as with the other ailments listed in this chapter and as with fibromyalgia itself.

Many people with GERD also have problems with insomnia, as do people with FMS. A low dose of an antidepressant may help resolve that problem. In the case of GERD, however, this advice is usually accompanied with other recommendations, such as to raise the head of the bed and to avoid late-night eating. Exercising and weight loss are also common recommendations given to people with chronic heartburn.

If you have more than one illness, you may receive medications for each medical problem. The situation can be further complicated when you see more than one doctor, particularly if you make the bad mistake of not telling each doctor about every single medication you take, including all vitamins and supplements, as well as all prescribed drugs. Each drug that you take has the potential to change the effect of every other drug. It may boost or weaken the effects of other medications or change their effects in some other way. Some drug interactions can be dangerous.

Dealing with depression

If you have fibromyalgia, you're also at risk for depression. *Depression* is a severely low mood state, in which a person has feelings of poor self-worth, appetite and sleep disturbances, and a loss of enjoyment in activities that used to be pleasurable. It's more pronounced and longer lasting than a temporary state of sadness. At worst, the depressed person considers or acts on suicidal thoughts. At "best," the person feels sad and distressed. Thankfully, though, depression is highly treatable.

Diagnosing depression

Many primary care physicians can recognize and treat depression, although they may want to refer the patient to a *psychiatrist*, a specialist in treating emotional disorders.

One problem that some people with fibromyalgia face is that doctors (not just psychiatrists) may see the depression as the entire problem rather than one piece of the fibromyalgia symptoms puzzle. Thus, if the depression is treated, then the mood disorder may lift, but the pain, fatigue, and other symptoms of the fibromyalgia may continue on as before, unabated and unrelenting. If you feel like you're being shuttled off to a shrink when you urgently need help for your pain, maybe you're right. Speak up for yourself.

Treating depression with medication or therapy

Depressive disorders are usually treated with antidepressant drugs and therapy. Doctors have many different types of antidepressant medications to choose from. If a drug from one category doesn't work, another medication may be effective.

The older and less expensive antidepressant drugs such as Elavil may also be useful in treating pain syndromes; consequently, the patient may obtain the impact of "two for the price of one" if she takes such a drug.

Depression is often treated effectively by therapists using *cognitive-behavioral therapy* (CBT), which is sometimes known simplistically as "talk therapy." With this therapy, the therapist teaches the person to realize and analyze *how* they're thinking about their problems. (That's the "cognitive" part.) The therapist using CBT then shows patients how they can challenge their own erroneous assumptions — the "behavioral" part of CBT. For example, if you think or fear that you have fibromyalgia because you're a bad person, and, consequently, you somehow deserve to be sick, then you're unlikely to take any sustained action that could help you feel better.

The CBT therapist can help you identify underlying mistaken or ill-serving assumptions about yourself (which you may never have challenged or even noticed before), replacing them with better ones. Such as replacing negative, self-abasing thoughts with something like this: "I do *not* deserve to have this medical problem, and I *can* feel better! And I really deserve to be well!"

Then you can subsequently work toward finding and implementing effective ways to help you work toward your own much-deserved wellness. I have many ideas in this book for you to try in order to reach that important goal!

Chapter 3

Understanding Possible Causes of Fibromyalgia

- -

- -

*L*isa was in a very bad car crash; the air bag was released so explosively that powder from the air bag flew under her contact lenses and temporarily damaged her eyes. She recovered from the accident, or thought she did, but then Lisa began suffering from severe and widespread pain and fatigue. Her symptoms continued to baffle her doctors for several years before one of them finally diagnosed her with fibromyalgia.

Jamie, on the other hand, has had no accidental injuries, and she really can't trace the onset of her fibromyalgia. In fact, she says that she doesn't know when she did *not* have the symptoms of fibromyalgia. As long as she can remember, she's suffered from pain, fatigue, and *brain fog* (memory problems and confusion associated with fibromyalgia). Jamie has forgotten exactly how many doctors she may have seen before her condition was finally diagnosed. She does know her sister, mother, and aunt also have very similar symptoms, and she's urged them to ask their doctors if they could have fibromyalgia, too. Jamie believes that fibromyalgia has a genetic basis because it seems to run in her family.

Both Lisa and Jamie have fibromyalgia syndrome (FMS), although the probable causes for each woman's current condition are apparently different. A trauma to the body can sometimes cause a long-term effect that translates into fibromyalgia, as in Lisa's case. And some people may have a genetic predisposition to developing fibromyalgia, as Jamie believes. Her belief that her family members have FMS may not be right, but she *is* right in actively urging them to obtain the medical help that they need.

From injuries and other forms of physical trauma to infections, environmental causes and the effects of genetics, I discuss the primary causes for why people develop fibromyalgia in this chapter.

What is for Certain About Fibromyalgia

Research has shown that fibromyalgia can be triggered by injuries (especially neck injuries), infections, and traumatic events. So I begin this chapter discussing these causes, moving afterward to more speculative causes for fibromyalgia, such as environmental causes, Gulf War syndrome, chemical imbalances, immune problems, and other causes. However, I can't tell you which single cause is the "right" one for all people. In fact, fibromyalgia probably doesn't have one single cause; it may instead have multiple causes.

I can tell you that research is ongoing and will hopefully bring us the keys to unlocking the underlying causes of this syndrome. Discovery is an ongoing process. Hey, who knew that mold (which we use for penicillin to fight infections) would actually be good for you? Science continues to march forward, sometimes lurching sideways to make unexpected new findings that help us.

Down But Not Out: Physical Trauma

A physical trauma may be traumatic enough for some people to ultimately develop FMS. In addition to an accidental injury, some researchers have argued that the onset of fibromyalgia can be attributed to previous physical or sexual abuse.

In these cases of fibromyalgia, the people were basically healthy before the injuries occurred, and they had no or few symptoms of fibromyalgia. However, at some point after the accidental injury or trauma, fibromyalgia moved in and seemed to make a permanent home for itself in their bodies.

Although current studies seem to indicate a relationship of FMS with a previous trauma, future large, prospective studies need to be conducted to definitively prove this relationship.

Looking at types of trauma that may cause FMS

What kinds of physical trauma may trigger fibromyalgia? The syndrome can result from an injury due to a car crash, or it may stem from a serious accidental injury that happened at work. Even a major fall can be enough to produce the symptoms of fibromyalgia in some people. For other individuals, a medical crisis may trigger the development of FMS. A medical crisis is something like a severe infection, surgery, or a diabetic crisis. No one knows how often severe traumas actually lead to the development of fibromyalgia, but probably no more than half (at most) of all cases of FMS stem from physical trauma.

Severe accidental injuries

Debbie was in a car crash, and although she didn't break any bones, she had a great deal of soft tissue damage. She says that she was covered from head to toe with bruises. After the accident, Debbie began experiencing severe headaches and extreme overall pain. She had been a successful computer programmer, but she had to ultimately give up her much-loved programming career. Debbie says that she couldn't write programs anymore, and she couldn't even *read* or comprehend what was on the computer screen most of the time, nor could she make sense of written instructions off the screen. She struggled, and mostly failed, to stay on task because of so much difficulty with reading instructions and remembering what she was doing.

Rebecca, another person whose FMS apparently stemmed from a physical trauma, began experiencing fibromyalgia pain and symptoms after a very bad fall. She slipped and fell, breaking her leg, heel, and toes. In addition to the FMS symptoms, she developed very severe pain in her knee, which her doctors diagnosed as arthritis. Following the advice of her doctors, Rebecca had a knee reconstruction. Her knee felt better after the surgery, but her overall body pain then began in earnest.

Rebecca says that she had enormous trouble sleeping, and, at best, she was clocking three or four hours of sleep per night. She also had trouble walking around. Sometimes these difficulties became extreme, and Rebecca says that she had to go to the hospital emergency room 12 times in 1999.

Rebecca was finally diagnosed with fibromyalgia in 2001 by a doctor who actually listened to her symptoms, performed a thorough physical examination, ordered laboratory tests to rule out other illnesses, and then correctly deduced that the problem was fibromyalgia (probably caused by the fall) and began to treat it.

Physical or sexual abuse

Physical abuse is another type of trauma that may lead to fibromyalgia. Some people were subjected to physical or sexual abuse during their childhood. Jeanne calls herself an "incest survivor" because a family member sexually abused her when she was a little girl. Jeanne says that she also suffered from stress that stemmed from the abuse, and she later developed fibromyalgia as well.

In another case, Sara, who was physically abused by her husband, says that various doctors have suspected that her fibromyalgia was triggered by a near-death beating during which she also suffered a serious head injury and neck trauma.

Some people who were abused as children continue to be abused as adults by their spouses or other individuals. All that physical battering can eventually take its painful toll on the human body, and sometimes the "price" is fibromyalgia.

Because of these associations, your doctor may ask you probing questions pertaining to sensitive areas of your personal life, including abusive relationships, sexual abuse, or physical trauma. Try not to be offended but rather understand that she's merely trying to understand your clinical situation more clearly. Seeking treatment and counseling for these contributing factors may be as important in your therapy as any medicinal treatments.

Extreme life-threatening illness

Tammy says that she was fine until, for some reason, she developed a serious brain aneurysm that burst and required emergency surgery. Fortunately, the brain surgery was successful — or so she thought. But shortly afterwards, Tammy began experiencing severe fatigue, muscle aches, a hard knot at the top of her left shoulder, and other symptoms — all of which were later diagnosed as fibromyalgia. Since then, she has wondered whether this trauma may somehow have triggered or unmasked her fibromyalgia.

Tammy's illness is an example of how physical trauma to the body, including from an extremely severe medical condition, can be a shock that precipitates the development of fibromyalgia. Long after the cause of the illness, such as Tammy's brain aneurysm, has passed, the effects of the trauma remain and must be dealt with.

Injuring yourself on the job

Could your symptoms stem from a work injury? A *repetitive strain injury,* or an injury that stems from repeated motions, such as from work on an assembly line, may trigger the development of fibromyalgia. (The most commonly known repetitive strain injury is *carpal tunnel syndrome*, which is damage to a nerve in the hand that results from repeated motions.) An accidental injury at work may also cause fibromyalgia.

If you think that your fibromyalgia may stem from an injury that occurred while you were at work or as a result of the work that you perform, you may be eligible for worker's compensation. In a precedent-setting 1999 Illinois case (*Waldorf Corporation versus Industrial Commission*), a worker whose job was to stack cartons in repetitive motions was diagnosed by a rheumatologist with fibromyalgia, and she sought worker's compensation. She won at the lower level, but the case was appealed by her employer. The worker was upheld. (Read more about work and fibromyalgia in Chapter 17.)

Other traumas

Even a very difficult pregnancy may trigger fibromyalgia in some susceptible people. Rose says that she was always a sickly child with FMS-like problems, but her really major symptoms didn't develop until she became pregnant. After that, she became increasingly ill until finally, to her great dismay, Rose became completely bedridden with fibromyalgia when her daughter was about 6 years old. Her case is a severe one. Most people don't become this disabled from fibromyalgia.

Investigating how physical trauma can trigger FMS

No one knows for sure how physical trauma or abuse can trigger fibromyalgia. But what may happen is that the body's stress response is shocked. The stress response system may rush to help the body resist the trauma by mobilizing *hormones* (chemicals created by the body, such as thyroid hormone, cortisol, and adrenalin) and *neurochemicals* (chemicals created by the brain, such as serotonin or dopamine). The body may hyper-react to extreme trauma, to the extent that, when the incident is over, the reactions continue on.

For example, imagine your body as a sort of living house. Intruders break into the house and attack it. They smash the windows and slash the carpet. They throw paint on the walls. If a house were alive, it would try to repair itself after the attack ended and the intruders were gone. It would also be vigilant. If the house could somehow give itself burglar alarms and a security system, it would do so.

Imagine if the live "house" decided to *really* protect itself from any future attacks, by surrounding itself with razor wire, armed guards with machine guns, and killer dogs. This protection would be an overreaction, just as sometimes after a trauma, people's bodies go into a hypersensitive and over reactive mode, too.

Post-traumatic stress disorder and FMS

Unusual stress and trauma possibly may trigger Fibromyalgia after an extremely distressing event. This reaction is known as *post-traumatic stress disorder (PTSD)*. The body apparently goes into a hyper-aroused state, and the individual may suffer from extreme anxiety that continues long after the distressing incident occurred. People who suffer from PTSD can develop physical symptoms that lead to fibromyalgia soon after the incident or after six months or more.

PTSD may be caused by such horrors as witnessing the violent death of another person, experiencing rape or severe physical abuse, or being threatened with death. Other causes are torture, natural disasters, severe car crashes, or being told that one has a life-threatening illness. The person who suffers from PTSD typically re-experiences the event in their minds, including the anguish and pain they felt when it actually happened. The person with PTSD also usually actively seeks to avoid anything that may remind him or her of the terrifying incident,

including people or places associated with it. PTSD affects a person's performance at work and their social functioning.

PTSD has some basic symptoms, according to the *Diagnostic and Statistical Manual of Mental Disorders, DSM-IV-TR* (a book used by mental health professionals), published by the American Psychiatric Association. When a person has PTSD, the following symptoms become present and were *not* there before the traumatic incident:

✔ Sleep disorders, such as trouble falling asleep or frequent awakenings

✔ Angry or irritable outbursts

✔ Problems with concentration

✔ *Hypervigilance:* Always on the watch for danger to appear on the horizon. The person has an extreme startle response. Someone touches him unexpectedly, and he jerks far more violently than normal.

Catching FMS

Some experts have hypothesized that fibromyalgia may result from a bacterial or viral infection, which triggers the FMS symptoms. In some cases, the infection may cause the immune system to go into hyperdrive. Research has borne out that infections can trigger the development of fibromyalgia in some people.

In a study reported in a 2001 issue of the *Journal of Rheumatology*, Danish researchers compared the presence of antibodies (chemicals the body created to kill invading bacteria or viruses) to *enterovirus* (a common viral infection) in 19 people with an acute onset of fibromyalgia to 20 subjects with a slow onset of FMS. They found that half the people with a sudden onset of FMS tested positive for the antibodies, but only 15 percent of the subjects with a slow onset of fibromyalgia had the antibodies in their systems. Based on these results, the researchers concluded that some patients with fibromyalgia may have different immune responses. Although this theory may sound far fetched, it's certainly possible.

After all, for many years, most doctors around the entire globe believed that ulcers were primarily caused by high levels of stress. Yet in 1982, two Australian doctors insisted that most ulcers were actually caused by bacteria. These doctors were ignored or ridiculed mercilessly by most of the global medical community. But finally in 1994, the National Institutes of Health, which had tested and proven the bacterial theory, acknowledged that most ulcers are, indeed, caused by *Helicobacter pylori*, a common form of bacteria found worldwide.

The point here is not what causes ulcers but instead is this: Just because we don't *know* if bacteria or virus can cause FMS doesn't mean that they *don't* cause it. Some preliminary pharmaceutical research with *interferon*, a human immunity-boosting chemical, has demonstrated that some people with FMS respond well to the drug, indicating that an immune system problem may be at work in at least a portion of the people who have fibromyalgia. (Read Chapter 10 for more information on current and developing medications to treat fibromyalgia.)

Interestingly, some people have an immune system that apparently goes into hyperdrive, turning on itself. This is called an *autoimmune reaction,* and it may be a cause of fibromyalgia. Conversely, other people may have lethargic immune systems that are basically run-down. Both paths may lead to "Fibromyalgia Land."

From a viral infection

Carla says that a virus may have triggered her fibromyalgia. She was very healthy until she came down with a severe mosquito-borne virus that she contracted in Australia. At the same time, her marriage failed, and she faced extreme stress from that breakup. The physical and emotional factors, together with the damage to her body caused by the infection, may have thrown Carla's entire body into a turmoil, or so her doctors have hypothesized.

In another case, Janet's fibromyalgia symptoms began several months after she'd recovered from a bout with mononucleosis, which may have triggered her FMS.

For both Carla and Janet, an infection appears to have played a role in the development of their FMS. Thus, indirectly, their fibromyalgia was "catching."

From an autoimmune reaction

It may also be possible that an FMS sufferer had an actual infection to the body, but that person's body hyper-reacted to the bacterial or viral invader by creating an excessive response of the immune system, generating high levels of antibodies. Those high levels of antibodies may have continued to act well after they were still needed, leading to the damaging condition we know as fibromyalgia.

This theory makes particular sense, especially when considering that many people with already-diagnosed autoimmune disease, such as lupus, may also suffer from a form of fibromyalgia. Therefore, all people being diagnosed with fibromyalgia should have an evaluation to make sure that they don't have a recognized autoimmune disorder precipitating their symptoms.

Honing in on hepatitis C

Other infectious diseases have been associated with fibromyalgia; for example, in a study reported in a 1997 issue of the *British Journal of Rheumatology*, the researchers found that 17 fibromyalgia patients (15 percent of their subjects with FMS) tested positive for having antibodies from hepatitis C. *Hepatitis C* is an infectious disease that attacks the liver. It is transmitted through body fluids.

As a result of their study, the researchers recommended that physicians who suspect that their patients may have fibromyalgia should rule out hepatitis C as a possible cause of the medical problem. If hepatitis C is found, the disease (hepatitis C) can be treated with the appropriate medications (such as inter-feron and *ribavirin*, an antiviral drug) as well as with other recommendations the physician may have.

This evidence doesn't mean that everyone or even most people with fibromyalgia have hepatitis C. Instead, it means that hepatitis C may cause fibromyalgia-like symptoms, and, thus, hepatitis C may need to be ruled out as the cause of these symptoms. This need for testing is particularly true if the individual experienced a blood transfusion before 1990. (After 1990, test-ing to screen for hepatitis C was developed.) Testing is also necessary if the individual has injected illegal drugs because hepatitis C is transmitted through the blood.

From other infections

Some experts say that some patients with fibromyalgia may have been previously infected with viruses such as the *Epstein-Barr virus* (a common virus that causes infectious mononucleosis), or with *Lyme disease*, a tick-borne illness that was originally discovered in Lyme, Connecticut. In the case of Lyme disease patients who develop FMS, their fibromyalgia symptoms typically don't improve with the normal antibiotic regimen that's prescribed for Lyme disease. The causal relationship of these infections with FMS, however, is still unproved.

Regarding Gulf War Syndrome

After the Gulf War in 1991, similar to many other military campaigns, as many as half of the military people who had recently served in the Persian Gulf reported suffering from symptoms of muscle pain, headaches, difficulty with memory, and fatigue. Among their military compatriots who did *not* serve in the Gulf War region during the same time frame, only about 15 percent reported similar complaints. In retrospect, many of the veterans' complaints, also generically known as "Gulf War syndrome," may have been consistent with a diagnosis of fibromyalgia. However, despite intensive research, no one could find any specific environmental agents that would explain the Gulf veterans' symptoms.

Some researchers have speculated that the military people who served in the Gulf during the war may have contracted a viral or bacterial infection that could have led to their symptoms, perhaps one that was further aggravated by the heightened stress of undergoing warfare in another country. Others think that severe stress alone could have been sufficient to induce the medical problems that the veterans suffered from.

In one study of Gulf War veterans (104 men and 21 women) who complained of a variety of symptoms, the researchers at Oregon Health Sciences University in Portland, Oregon found that 27 percent of the veterans met the criteria for chronic fatigue syndrome and 14 percent met the diagnostic criteria for fibromyalgia.

Honing in on hormonal changes to the vets

The researchers also found that the veterans with fibromyalgia had low levels of growth hormone, a hormone that works to repair muscle tissue. Some civilians diagnosed with fibromyalgia had been found to have similarly low levels of this same hormone.

Researchers say that stress can inhibit the production of growth hormones. So, perhaps the military veterans who were in a state of heightened stress under war conditions produced less growth hormone, which then led to the development of fibromyalgia. This theory remains unproved, but it's an intriguing possible explanation for a higher than normal incidence of fibromyalgia among military veterans who served in the Gulf War.

Actions that can make fibromyalgia worse

This chapter focuses on possible *causes* of fibromyalgia, but you should also know some basics about what can aggravate an existing case of FMS in many people. So here's a quick list of watch-out-for items for you to consider:

✔ **Consuming copious quantities of alcohol:** You may think that alcohol will help you fall asleep. The reality is that you may pass out from drinking, but you'll usually wake up in the middle of the night feeling awful. (Read more about alcohol and fibromyalgia in Chapter 15.)

✔ **Staying up very late and skimping on your sleep time:** In fact, some experts believe that inadequate sleep can actually *cause* FMS, not just worsen it. (When you read Chapter 14, you find out why sleep deprivation is so bad. But the short answer is that inadequate sleep can *really* worsen existing fibromyalgia for most people.)

✔ **Stressing out in a major way about your personal, work, or family problems:** Stressing out on just about anything, in fact, can really aggravate your symptoms, making it important for FMS sufferers to figure out how to relax. (Read more about "depressurizing" yourself in Chapter 13.)

✔ **Eating only junk food, like soda, chocolate candy, and sugary substances:** Ouch! You're going to regret it when the pain kicks in. (Chapter 15 offers good advice on good foods and bad foods.)

✔ **Experiencing changing weather conditions:** You can't wish the bad weather away, but at least you can anticipate its effects on you. (See Chapter 2 for more information on weather sensitivity.)

Not a new problem

Unexplained musculoskeletal pain, fatigue, and sleep problems have been observed after every military conflict as far back as the Civil War. To date, researchers haven't been able to identify any specific environmental agent as the cause or the trigger of the particular symptoms experienced by the veterans. The one thing they *do* all have in common is the stress that occurs during war times.

Helping Gulf War veterans

No one may be able to explain why veterans return from war with symptoms of chronic illnesses, but that doesn't mean that these veterans can't get help. Veterans who served in the Gulf and who have since been diagnosed with chronic illnesses — such as *chronic fatigue syndrome* (CFS), *irritable bowel syndrome* (IBS), or fibromyalgia — may be eligible and should apply for financial benefits that are available through the Veterans Administration.

Congress passed a law in 1994 to cover military veterans with symptoms of medical problems, such as chronic fatigue syndrome and fibromyalgia, but many veterans were denied benefits. In January of 2002, a new law was passed to broaden the coverage to more veterans of the Gulf War (Public Act 107-103). The application deadline for these benefits is September 30, 2011. About 3,200 veterans were approved for compensation prior to 2002, and it was estimated in 2002 that another 3,000 veterans would qualify for benefits under the new legislation. For further information, contact the nearest Veterans Administration office.

Studying Chemical Imbalances

Research has shown that, among people with fibromyalgia, some important body chemicals are significantly lower than normal, and others are significantly higher. This evidence may indicate that the problem is caused by a chemical imbalance. Some experts believe that the cause of these excessive or deficient levels of chemicals is due to a brain abnormality related to the interaction between important organs that regulate body chemicals, such as the hypothalamus, pituitary gland, and adrenal glands. What is generally accepted is that excessive or deficient levels of certain hormones from the hypothalamus, thyroid, pituitary, and adrenal glands could contribute to or cause fibromyalgia-type symptoms.

Impairments in these glands that cause deviations from the normal level of body chemicals can lead to troublesome difficulties with sleep, an increased risk for pain, and greater degrees of muscle pain, especially morning stiffness. They may also cause other symptoms that are commonly associated with fibromyalgia, such as fatigue and brain fog and it may worsen other medical conditions.

No one knows for sure what causes fibromyalgia, although a wide array of theories abound. Evidence is mounting, however, for profound central nervous system abnormalities in FMS. Whether fibromyalgia is just an extreme form of chronic musculoskeletal pain that, at normal levels, is very common in the general population needs to be determined. However, for people with fibromyalgia, speculating on *why* they've developed FMS — certainly an interesting topic — isn't as important as working with doctors on a good plan to minimize the pain, fatigue, and other symptoms.

Substance P = Pain

Substance P is a brain/pain neurochemical with the main purpose of sending pain messages to the body. "It's time to hurt! Say 'ouch!'" Normally, this pain message isn't a bad thing because people *need* to feel pain when they experience harm, so that they can take the appropriate action to resolve the situation. The problem with fibromyalgia, however, is that the pain signal the individual feels is way out of proportion to minor injuries or illnesses. (Read more about pain in Chapter 4.)

Researchers have demonstrated that people with FMS generate abnormally high levels of Substance P. In fact, studies have shown that some people with fibromyalgia have as much as three times the levels of Substance P in their cerebrospinal fluid (a special fluid found in your backbone) than is found in people who don't have fibromyalgia.

Experts don't know whether excessive levels of Substance P are the *cause* of fibromyalgia symptoms or the *result* of them. And, actually, experts don't even know *if* Substance P is the cause or the result of FMS at all. The high amount of Substance P could just be a byproduct of other biochemical processes. (Yes, I know that trying to categorize the cause of this elusive fibromyalgia syndrome can be very frustrating, sort of like trying to nail down mercury or gelatin. Just when you think you have it, it slips away.)

Everyone's body releases some amount of Substance P as a normal course of events when painful stimuli occur. But you certainly don't want to have excessive levels of Substance P in your body. Unfortunately, you can't flip a "halfway" or a "low" switch in your brain like you would adjust a thermostat up or down to scale things down if your body is churning out too much of this chemical. Your brain's control panel is currently inaccessible.

Instead, medications and treatments must be used to counteract the effects of Substance P and the accompanying array of symptoms that are associated with fibromyalgia.

Neurochemically affecting your pain/symptomatic levels

Some studies of people with fibromyalgia have indicated other neurochemicals, in addition to Substance P, as possible causes or contributors to the problem. Thyroid hormone is a critically important hormone that regulates the body's energy expenditure and metabolism. Some people who suffer from chronic fatigue, wide-ranging muscle pain, and sleep disturbances are ultimately found to have elevated or depressed levels of circulating thyroid hormone. This can occur for many reasons but, in most instances, can be appropriately controlled, leading to improvement in symptoms. Cortisol is an important hormone that's secreted by the adrenal glands. It maintains blood pressure, blood sugar, and other important biological functions that help people cope with stress. Studies indicate that some people with FMS have inadequate levels of cortisol in the daytime (making them feel fatigued) and then too much cortisol at night (causing insomnia).

People with fibromyalgia sometimes experience below-normal levels of brain chemicals, such as *serotonin*, a calming brain chemical. Also, some people with fibromyalgia have below-normal levels of growth hormones, which are hormones that even adults have that perform basic repair work at the cellular level. Insufficient growth-hormone levels may mean that damaged cells stay damaged longer, causing pain and other symptoms.

Examining Environmental Causes

Maybe it's an allergy that some people's bodies react to quite extremely or it could be a substance that some people consume and react negatively to. Doctors don't know for sure, so the studies continue.

Considering an allergic reaction

Another theory about FMS is that it may result from the body's allergic reaction to something else in the environment, whether it's chemicals, smoke, or other irritants. This may be why antihistamines can make some people with fibromyalgia feel better — the antihistamine drugs quell the action of the body's *histamines*, which are chemicals released by the body when confronted with an allergic agent.

Experiencing a hypersensitivity to chemicals

Some people may be overly sensitive to many chemicals in their environ-ment. Most people in the United States are constantly exposed to a barrage of chemicals, but their bodies can usually cope with them. However, some people may go into a sort of "systems overload." They don't actually die, but their bodies react so strongly that it may lead to the pain, sleep difficulties, muscular stiffness, and other problems that are characteristic of fibromyal-gia. Some people respond very severely to cigarette smoke, perfumes, and industrial chemicals.

Feeling the effects of phosphates

Some people are convinced that people with fibromyalgia build up storage areas of chemicals in their bodies that clog up their systems with substances that the kidneys are unable to excrete fast enough. They see the primary culprit as a series of numerous, heavy deposits of *phosphates* — chemicals stemming from products containing the element of phosphorus. The theory is that salicylate generates phosphates; including aspirin itself, as well as topical ointments containing aspirin and other products. This is why *guaifenesin* has been advocated to help break up the phosphates that are supposedly present. Guaifenesin is a drug that's available in both prescribed and over-the-counter dosages, which is normally taken to treat coughs.

Guaifenesin users believe that doses of this medication can eventually alleviate the pain, fatigue, and other symptoms of FMS, although clinical studies have yet to bear them out. (Read more about the use of guaifenesin in treating fibromyalgia in Chapter 9.)

Suffering from hyper-arousability

Some people with fibromyalgia, for whatever reason (hormonal, viral, or something else), become extremely sensitive to loud noises, strong light, and other stimuli. Carol says that she stopped sleeping with her husband because he snores. So, now, she sleeps in another room with a big blanket over the closed window to keep out the noise and the light. Carol also got rid of a ticking clock in the room, whose noise she says drove her "wild." Her children call Carol's new bedroom her "sensory deprivation room." Carol says spending time in this room makes her feel much better. And it certainly enables her to sleep better.

It's almost as if Carol, as well as some others who have fibromyalgia, has lost some of her basic sensory screening-out abilities. Or perhaps she and others with FMS are too highly sensitive. Either way, they feel nearly as overstimulated as a person suffering from *autism*, a disorder in which the individual feels completely bombarded with stimuli, even in a low-key situation. The slightest touch, sound, or other stimulus causes irritation, and as the stimulus increases in intensity, it causes physical pain.

Exploring Other Theories

Other theories also try to explain why fibromyalgia strikes some people and not others. For example, maybe it's in the genes, and you inherit this propensity from your parents. Or, FMS may result from too much or too little exercising. Fibromyalgia may also be caused by a structural defect at the cellular level. I explore all these possibilities in the following sections.

Linking genetics and fibromyalgia

Can something in your genes cause fibromyalgia? Can you really inherit the risk for developing fibromyalgia if other people in your family are diagnosed with the syndrome? Based on the reports of most FMS sufferers, fibromyalgia seems to "run in" families. And many medical problems have a genetic basis.

Today, many doctors believe that numerous people may have a genetic predisposition to a wide variety of different medical problems; however, something in the environment (contracting a virus, being involved in a car crash, or facing other types of severe trauma to the body) may have to actually trigger this predisposition to developing fibromyalgia or other medical problems.

Doctors and researchers are working very hard to map the human genetic codes and to try to determine which genes weaken the body and lead to medical problems and which ones work to protect the body and prevent serious illnesses. But the genetic link (if one even exists) is still unknown.

Despite this lack of evidence, many people are still convinced that fibromyalgia must be a hereditary medical problem. For example, Denise says that she has always had fibromyalgia symptoms, and her mother and her two sisters have them as well. The symptoms flare up when they become very stressed out and upset. But Denise is the only family member who has been diagnosed with fibromyalgia so far. Denise has three children, and two of them — teenage girls, ages 14 and 16 — have the very same overall painful symptoms that Denise and her sisters suffer from. Denise thought her daughters were too young to have fibromyalgia, but she's rethinking her position and plans to take the girls in for medical evaluations.

A shared environment

One potential problem with the genetic-cause theory is that people in nuclear families (adults and children, usually two generations) generally also have a shared environment. Because they live together and are in close contact with each other, they come down with the same viruses and are exposed to the same chemicals. They eat the same foods. They also share the same lifestyle — for example, being very active or more on the sedentary side. As a result, if more than one family member has fibromyalgia, the medical problem may actually derive from some undefined element from within their shared environment, rather than from a shared gene pool.

Analyzing your family tree: What to ask

In attempting to determine whether members of your extended family (primarily your parents and siblings) have fibromyalgia, too, it's best to avoid asking them if they have FMS. They may never have heard of it. Instead, ask them if they frequently have lots of pain, particularly around the neck, shoulders, and back areas. Keep in mind that older relatives (over age 65) may have pain in those areas, but it could be pain that's also associated with arthritis.

Then, ask about any problems with continuous and severe fatigue. If you receive another "yes," continue on with the other symptoms of fibromyalgia, such as sleep problems, chronic headaches, irritable bowel syndrome, and so forth. Do not, however, announce to your relatives who seem to "qualify" that you *know* that they have fibromyalgia, even if they say "yes" to every symptom, and it seems glaringly obvious to you that, of course, they *must* have FMS. As discussed in Chapter 6, many medical conditions can be confused with fibromyalgia, and only a doctor can really determine if a person has FMS or not.

A research link

Dr. Muhammad B. Yunus at the University of Illinois College of Medicine in Peoria, Illinois, has studied 40 families with fibromyalgia and looked at possible hereditary factors at work. His research has found a weak correlation between the development of fibromyalgia in the *HLA allele,* a specific genetic location. Dr. Yunus and other researchers are continuing to look for specific genetic markers that may lead to the development of fibromyalgia among family members.

Looking at who is most at risk in your family

Because fibromyalgia is generally more prominently found among females than males, if FMS does actually "run" in families, you may expect to find it more frequently in your mother, aunts, grandmothers, sisters, and other female "blood" relatives rather than in your father, brothers, uncles, and other male relations. But keep an open mind. Men can have fibromyalgia, too, so it doesn't hurt to ask.

Even if practically everyone in your family seems to have all or most of the symptoms of fibromyalgia, this doesn't mean that you or your other relatives have FMS. And even if there *is* a genetic predisposition to FMS, this merely means that some people in the family may develop fibromyalgia, and others will not.

Exercising too little/too much

Some doctors and experts theorize that another underlying cause of fibromyalgia may be related to an extreme decrease or extreme increase in activity. Basically, this means that playing "couch potato" can transform a person into an unhappy fibromyalgiac. At the other end of the spectrum, a person can excessively exercise to the point that he or she has overstressed the body and inadvertently caused the onset of fibromyalgia symptoms.

In general, people with fibromyalgia have a lower pain threshold and a greater sensitivity to pain, and they also feel pain significantly longer than people who don't have fibromyalgia. What causes this hypersensitivity to pain is unclear, but it's apparent that this extreme pain sensitivity can impair a person's overall functioning, causing a negative downward spiral unless and until the cycle is broken. (Read Chapter 4 for more information on pain issues and fibromyalgia.)

As a result of this pain sensitivity, both under-exercising and over-exercising can worsen fibromyalgia pain. For example, Lethargic Lucy rarely exercises because it hurts too much. She's gotten very out of shape, which has caused her pain to worsen. At the other end of the spectrum, Dynamic Diana, an overly enthusiastic exerciser with fibromyalgia, is far more fit than Lethargic Lucy. But she's also more likely to incur injuries, along with the pain she incurs from excessive exercising. (Read Chapter 15 for important advice on exercise when you have FMS).

Considering muscular or structural abnormalities

Some researchers, using expensive high-tech electronic microscopes and other very specialized equipment, have studied tissue samples from people with fibromyalgia. They've found that FMS patients are more likely to have damaged muscle tissue than people who don't have fibromyalgia. Research continues on this high-tech front.

Suffering from a combo platter of illnesses

Maybe fibromyalgia results from a variety of different causes that interact with each other in a bad way. For example, perhaps some families have a genetic predisposition to an allergy. If that genetic propensity interacts with allergy-inducing substances, the result may be FMS. On the other hand, maybe some families have less effective immune systems, and its members are more at risk for contracting viruses and bacterial infections — and this combination may cause fibromyalgia. It may also be true that some families tend to have overactive immune systems, and their members are more at risk for experiencing a triggering of abnormal immune responses to viruses and bacterial infections, which may cause fibromyalgia.

Another possibility is that because of a highly stressful job, some people start to lose sleep on all or most nights. The sleep deprivation makes them feel worse. They may start overeating or consuming excessive amounts of alcohol to try to comfort themselves. The combination of events and personal decisions may cause or aggravate an active case of fibromyalgia.

Looking to the Future

You can drive yourself crazy trying to pin down the actual cause of fibromyalgia in yourself or other people. Research is actively ongoing, and I do anticipate many important breakthroughs in the near future.

For now, researchers and doctors can only theorize about what may cause fibromyalgia. We do know, however, that whatever the causes, fibromyalgia is a *real* syndrome that causes pain and suffering to millions of people, and it needs to be taken seriously.

Chapter 4

Understanding Fibromyalgia Pain

● ●

In This Chapter

▶ Recognizing that pain has both bad and good (really!) roles in life

▶ Seeing how fibromyalgia pain is different from non-fibromyalgia pain

▶ Understanding that all pain can't be eliminated — nor should it be

▶ Discovering what pain management is and how it can help

▶ Keeping a pain/symptom diary

● ●

*P*ain is bad. But pain is also good. And yes, these seemingly contradictory statements are both true. I know that the idea of pain as a useful thing is very hard to wrap your mind around when you're suffering from frequent and severe pain. And yet, gaining an understanding of both the pros and cons of pain is important. Why? Because knowledge is one giant step towards mastery. And wouldn't you like to be *more* in charge of your fibromyalgia pain?

The main problem with fibromyalgia is that it's pain run amuck, like the proverbial headless chicken. Another problem with fibromyalgia syndrome (FMS) is that chronic and sustained pain, such as the kind that many people with fibromyalgia most frequently experience, can be very bad for the body. The key with fibromyalgia pain is to control it, keeping it from a scream to a whisper.

In this chapter, I describe the purpose of pain — and it really does have a purpose (actually, more than one). I also talk about pain management and its importance. You may not (and usually can't) succeed at wiping out all your fibromyalgia pain forever. But you can tame it from a raging wild stallion to a sort of gentle nag, and, in most cases, you can also lead a far more normal life than you may be experiencing right now.

Grasping Pain and Why People Have to Have It

If you have fibromyalgia, you know what pain is because you feel it probably every day and at differing levels of intensity. You'd probably like to "grasp" your fibromyalgia pain and throw it out the window forever. But before you explore ways to get rid of pain, you first need to understand pain: what it is and why you feel it.

Pain defined

Pain (mild to severe discomfort stemming from an injury, an illness, or from unknown sources) comes from one of two types of stimuli:

- **An outside stimulus:** The "Ouch! That hurts!" pain response from a paper cut, for example.
- **An internal stimulus:** Tightened muscles, for example.

Pain can be chronic or acute:

- *Acute pain* is pain that's always temporary.
- *Chronic pain* is pain that is sometimes worse and sometimes better, but it's basically always hanging around at some level.

With fibromyalgia, whatever caused the initial trauma to the body — whether it was an outside stimulus, such as an accidental injury, or an internal stimulus, such as a virus or something else altogether — the pain is chronic.

Its advantages and disadvantages

I know it's hard to believe, but pain plays a crucial and good role in your life. Here are the primary advantages of pain to human bodies:

- **Pain provides an early warning system of harm to the body and helps you detect damage or medical problems before they get out of control.** For example, if you have pain with urination, this pain may indicate a bladder infection. If you have chronic headaches, the cause may be sinusitis or a more serious medical problem. If you have constant pain after eating, you may have chronic heartburn or another medical condition. In each of these cases, your pain warns you to see your doctor for further evaluation. Without pain, a medical problem can worsen without your knowledge.

✔ **Pain enables us to take action now to stop the pain.** Of course, you can't go rushing off to the doctor every time you have a minor ache or pain. But if your pain is severe and/or chronic, your body is sending you a message. It's telling you that something is wrong. Do something about it right now! Ignoring your pain can be perilous to your health.

✔ **Pain allows us to prepare ahead and avoid worse pain.** When you know that something continues to bother you, with your physician's help, you can work on treating the problem and seek to identify patterns that seem to worsen the pain. Armed with that information, you can then avoid (or try to avoid) the painful stimulus in the future. For example, if you know that a bear hug is going to make you ache for days, based on the fact that it's happened before, you can warn people ahead of time that they really need to be gentle with you.

Pain can be very problematic, not only because pain *hurts* but also because it may lead to some long-term problems. In general, pain can be bad for your body for three main reasons:

✔ **Chronic pain wears down the body.** Like a truck spinning its wheels in the mud, smoke pouring from the engine, your body starts to break down under the added strain of chronic pain.

✔ **People who have chronic pain are prone to other illnesses.** Their immune systems may become weakened, and they may become more at risk for contracting the flu or whatever is the latest virus that's making the rounds among their family, friends, and coworkers. If you find yourself getting a strep throat and then the flu and then a bladder infection, you need your doctor's help to break out of this pattern. One way to break away is to accept that fact that chronic illness and pain are part of your problem, ask for help, and then to work on rebuilding your health.

✔ **Pain can harm your quality of life.** When pain is the pervasive influence in your life, you may find it hard to think about anything else or to achieve much of anything. When you're in severe pain, you may have trouble simply getting out of bed, let alone going to work to put in your eight or more hours. Pain also seeps into (or maybe floods into) other aspects of your life. For example, you can't help your child with her homework when you're overwhelmed with pain, nor can you pay attention to your partner or your friends.

Don't start doubting yourself when people say that they can't find anything wrong with you. Chronic pain is frequently undetectable. But the pain itself is always real. You don't feel chronic pain because you're upset or depressed or anxious or annoyed. You may be all those things — especially when people imply that your fibromyalgia pain is imaginary! But the pain itself is an independent and very real entity.

My pain studies on fibromyalgia

In 2000, I performed research at the University of Florida on volunteer patients, some of whom had fibromyalgia and some of whom did not, to determine whether the pain of FMS patients was somehow different from the pain experienced by people without fibromyalgia. My research revealed that the pain was both qualitatively and quantitatively different. What I mean is that for the people with fibromyalgia, the pain felt different, and they had a lot more of it.

I used mild heat stimulation and closely observed the reactions of the subjects. My study showed that the subjects *with* fibromyalgia felt pain sooner than the non-fibromyalgia subjects. Also,

their pain lasted significantly longer. I called that longer-lasting pain *windup pain*. What happens with most people who experience a mild pain is that they suffer briefly, and then the pain degrades and is soon gone. But people with fibromyalgia have an amplified pain that stays with them longer. It's almost as if the pain falls away from others like flakes of dust, but it somehow "sticks" for a longer time among people who have fibromyalgia.

With your doctor's help, you need to figure out what strategies and techniques can help you break out of this sustained pain syndrome, so that you can achieve major pain relief.

Regarding the Different Kind of Pain That's Fibromyalgia

Based on my research and the research of others, I can tell you that the pain that comes with fibromyalgia has three primary aspects. Very basically, people with fibromyalgia feel pain

- **Faster than others do:** FMS sufferers have a lowered pain threshold, meaning that, for example, if someone stuck a pin in you and another one in Susie (who doesn't have fibromyalgia), you'd probably yell before she would. (Read Chapter 3 for possible causes of this heightened pain.)

- **Worse than others do:** When you have fibromyalgia, you feel the pain more strongly. In fact, some tactile experiences that wouldn't bother Susie at all may really aggravate you. Some people with fibromyalgia say that when they're feeling bad, even something as normally benign as the cat rubbing up against them actually hurts.

- **For a longer time period than others do:** The pain keeps going and going and going, like the "Energizer Bunny" of pain. Suppose that Susie was pricked with a pin 20 minutes ago, and she's already forgotten about it and is outside raking leaves or talking on the phone with her friends. But you, with your fibromyalgia, are still sitting there, and you're still hurting.

Working with Your Doctor to Manage FMS Pain

Some pain can be cured permanently, but most chronic pain, such as the pain of FMS, can't be eradicated altogether and forever. Instead, the goal should be to manage FMS pain by radically decreasing it to a tolerable level. You can attain this goal through pain management. With the help of a good doctor (or two or more because, sometimes, you need the help of a specialist as well as your regular doctor), you can beat most pain into submission.

Pain management refers to all the actions that you and your doctor take to decrease (but usually not altogether eliminate), your fibromyalgia pain. It can be as simple an action as taking Tylenol or as complicated as combining medication with acupuncture, exercise, massage, and other options. The bottom line is that you were up at *here* (wherever that pain level was) when you started and then you go *down* to *here* (a lower level of pain) if the pain management has worked for you.

The best way to get pain relief is to work with a caring and knowledgeable doctor who listens to you and works to act in your best interests. And yes, such doctors are out there! If your doctor isn't helping you, you need to think about moving on to a doctor who *will* help you. (Read Chapter 7 for some help on finding a good doctor.)

Define your terms

The first step in managing the pain is to find out exactly how your doctor defines pain management. I know what *I* mean by pain management, but the term doesn't mean the same thing to all doctors. To one physician, pain management may mean that you're radically improved. To another, it means that you aren't calling him anymore; therefore, you must be better. And it has other meanings to other doctors.

Find out how your doctor defines pain management by asking the following questions:

- ✔ **Does pain management mean a cure?** In most cases, doctors will say "no." If the pain could be eliminated, it wouldn't need to be "managed." So, if the doctor says "yes," he can cure you, find another doctor.

- ✔ **Can most patients obtain some pain relief?** The right answer is nearly always "yes" Or something like "usually," or "in most cases." If the doctor says "no," you can't get any pain relief for your fibromyalgia, find another doctor.

> ✔ **What do you consider "success" in pain management?** It's impossible to evaluate here the many possible answers you may receive. Listen carefully and determine whether the doctor's answer makes sense to you.

After you and your doctor agree on what pain management is and what to expect from it, ask your doctor to help you formulate a plan to set you on the right path to managing your pain.

Plan a course of treatment

The doctor can't feel your pain, so she'll usually ask you how bad it is, on a scale of 1 to 10 — with 1 being minor pain and 10 being extremely severe pain. Once she knows how much pain you're in, she'll decide upon a course of action for you to try. Often she may prescribe medication, along with a hands-on therapy (such as heating or icing the painful area; both options are covered in Chapter 11).

Generally, the doctor will want you to follow her recommendations for a given period of time, which may be days or weeks, and will advise you to come back after that time for a follow-up visit. It's important to listen carefully to what your doctor recommends (it doesn't hurt to take notes!), and follow her instructions as closely as possible. If the recommendation doesn't work at all and your pain is still severe, tell the doctor, and she'll work on seeking other solutions for you.

Chart any changes

Part of working with your doctor is making sure that you report when you feel worse or when you feel better. Don't assume that your doctor somehow just knows that this new drug or treatment is great or terrible. Physicians are smart, but they aren't mind readers. Let them know about the bad and the good. If something helps you, it may help other people who are in fibromyalgia hell.

One way to help you track whether you're getting better, worse, or staying about the same is to document how you feel in a special diary. The reason for this diary is that you can very easily forget and think that you felt much worse (or maybe think you didn't feel that bad, when you did) if you don't keep a written record.

To help you keep track of how you feel, I've created a very simple pain and symptom diary for you to use (shown in Table 4-1). You can photocopy it or you can just copy the entries elsewhere. You don't need anything fancy — a simple student notebook would be fine. (For those of you who love computers, you can create a spreadsheet on the computer if you want, but it's certainly not necessary.)

Studies on women and pain

If you're a woman with fibromyalgia who thinks her pain may be undertreated, you may be right. In their article for a 2001 issue of the *Journal of Law, Medicine & Ethics*, authors Diane E. Hoffmann and Anita J. Tarzian analyzed studies of how men and women perceive pain as well as how their pain is regarded by doctors and nurses. The authors said that because women have pain more often than men and they are more pain sensitive, it would seem like they'd be treated by doctors at least as well as men are.

And yet, they aren't. Instead, women who report pain are *less* likely to be taken seriously and also less likely to receive adequate treatment for their pain.

Other researchers have shown that women experience fibromyalgia pain more and longer than men do. If you're a woman with fibromyalgia, don't let anyone tell you that your pain isn't real. Read more about women and fibromyalgia in Chapter 5.

You should try to make updates in your diary every day between visits to your doctor. At the end of each week, take a careful look at your pain diary to try to find patterns. Share your diary and any patterns that you notice with your doctor during your next visit.

I advise that you make entries in your pain diary even if you don't have any pain or much pain on one particular day, so that you'll have an accurate record. (Perhaps your pain management treatments are working. You'll want to record that.) You should also list any moderate to serious stress you faced, ranging from trouble at work or home to anything else that you know causes you to feel distressed.

Table 4-1	A Sample Pain and Symptom Diary						
	Mon	**Tues**	**Wed**	**Thurs**	**Fri**	**Sat**	**Sun**
Level of Pain (1–10)							
New treatments							
Stress							

As an example, say that Tina, who's been recently diagnosed with fibromyalgia, started keeping her own pain diary. Her first week's entries might look like the diary in Table 4-2.

As you can see from her chart, on Monday, Tina had severe pain at a level "9." That was also the day she started a new pain medication. On Tuesday, Tina had some pain but felt much better, and her pain was down to a "6." Nothing much else happened that day, so Tina wrote "no" for "new treatments" and "usual" for stress.

Then on Wednesday, Tina's pain went up a little to a "7." That was also the day her boss yelled at her, which she noted. Stress can increase pain, although it can't create it. Tina's pain was down to a "5" on Saturday but then went back up to a "7" on Sunday, when she was worried about her mother. All told, however, a "5" or a "6" is much better than her original "9" on the pain scale (which is where Tina started out), and consequently, the medication was a success.

Table 4-2		Tina's Pain/Symptom Diary					
	Mon	*Tues*	*Wed*	*Thurs*	*Fri*	*Sat*	*Sun*
Level of Pain (1–10):	9	6	7	5	5	5	7
New treatments:	Started new pain drug	No	No	Had massage	No	No	No
Stress:	Usual	Usual	Boss yelled	Usual	Usual	Easy day, rested	Mom sick, am worried

Move on to Plan B

Sometimes, when your doctor recommends a drug or a treatment, even if she's certain that this option is *the* most wonderful remedy on the planet, it just won't work for you. Give it a fair trial, though. Don't expect instant results from anything.

Some treatments may take days or weeks, and others may take months before you feel significantly better. How do you know how long is long enough before you should move on to Plan B and try something else? This decision really varies depending on the treatment. But to evaluate whether your pain management is having a significant effect, consider these points:

✔ Have you followed the doctor's recommendations or treatments? If the doctor told you to take a medication daily for a month and you took it once or twice, you didn't give it a fair trial.

✔ How long did the doctor tell you it would take for you to have any improvement? If the doctor said you'd feel better in days or weeks, and that time is past and your pain is unabated, it isn't working.

Are you a "painiac"?

If pain is completely dominating your life and it's also impairing your work and your relationships with others (as is the case for many people with fibromyalgia), you're probably also very distressed and upset much of the time. I've coined the very tongue-in-cheek term "painiac" to denote a person whose entire life is dominated by pain and its effects. Many people with fibromyalgia can easily slip into painiac status, but they shouldn't have to. They need to ask, or, if necessary, demand some help from their doctors.

Take this self-test to find out if you or someone you know can qualify as a painiac. Answer "true" or "false" to the following questions and then read further for an analysis of your answers.

- I turn down most invitations, including those to events I'd otherwise like to go to, because the pain is too great. Or I fear that it may become bad, so I don't want to go.

- If my child or someone I care about needs help with a project, I usually have to decline because of the pain.

- People say that I look normal, and don't understand how I can be hurting so much.

- I have few (or no) pain-free days.

- I have completely given up physical activities that I used to enjoy.

- Family members say that I'm the same person I was ten or more years ago.

Now, you need to analyze your answers. If you answered "true" to question 1, you've indicated that you may be at painiac status now. After the pain is under control, most people can return to socializing and other activities they like but that pain had stolen away from them.

In question 2, if you've had to say "no" when people you care about ask you for help, whether it's sewing a button on a shirt or asking you to read a term paper, because the pain was overwhelming you, you're at risk for painiac status.

Many people with fibromyalgia say that others remark on how "normal" they look, as in question 3. Because you're not gushing blood and your pain doesn't give any apparent visual cues, people find it hard to understand how you can be hurting so bad. If you feel like you're receiving this kind of feedback to your chronic pain, you're in danger of becoming a "painiac". (Read Chapter 16 for help on controlling your emotions.)

When you have very few (or maybe not *any*) pain-free days, as asked in question 4, your life is clearly dominated by pain. It's beyond time for you to step up to recognizing that you've got a problem here, and you need help. If your doctor can't or won't help you, you need to find another doctor. (Read Chapter 7 for help on identifying a good physician.)

If you've given up most activities that you enjoy, as asked in question 5, you're at risk for becoming a "painiac". Talk to your doctor about it and ask for help.

If family members say that you're just the same person you always were, as asked in question 6, they may be fibbing, or maybe your fibromyalgia isn't that bad. Or maybe you've been sick so long that it's the only way people see you. But for most readers, the answer to this question is "false."

Sometimes, people with fibromyalgia (or their doctors) attribute virtually any pain to their fibromyalgia. Your head hurts, and you think it's your fibromyalgia. Your back acts up; it's that pesky fibromyalgia again. Your toe aches, so it must be fibromyalgia. But people with FMS can have pain from problems other than fibromyalgia. If any of the following occurs, contact your doctor right away because these problems may indicate a medical condition that has nothing to do with your FMS:

✔ The pain is sudden and far more extreme than it has ever been before.

✔ The pain is accompanied by symptoms that you haven't seen before, such as dizziness, racing pulse, weakness, or mental confusion.

✔ You experience bleeding or visible body changes, such as extreme paleness or redness.

Part II
Finding Out If You Have Fibromyalgia

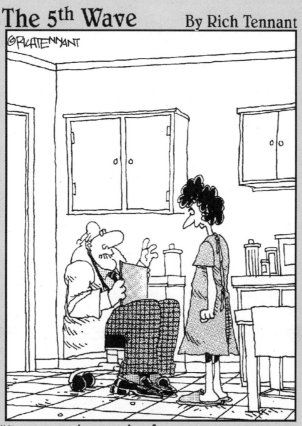

The 5th Wave   By Rich Tennant

"I was just surprised you put the word 'Marriage' next to the question asking if you suffered from a chronic condition."

In this part . . .

*I*f you think that you're the only person who has
fibromyalgia, well, think again! About 6 million people
in the United States and millions more worldwide know
exactly what you're going through. Who *are* these people?
I'm glad you asked that question because that's the subject of Chapter 5, where I describe the patterns found
among people most likely to suffer from fibromyalgia.

Part II is about finding out if *you* have fibromyalgia, and
part of that process is ruling out other medical problems
that may be impostors for your real problem of fibromyalgia. These conditions include chronic fatigue syndrome,
myofascial pain syndrome, arthritis, thyroid disease, and
a few other illnesses that may surprise you, such as Lyme
disease (all discussed in Chapter 6). Then I move into the
diagnosis aspect of fibromyalgia. A good doctor is crucial
to managing fibromyalgia, and I discuss the important role
that doctors play in Chapter 7. I also offer advice on working with your regular doctor, and if that doesn't work, finding a new doc. Then I cover what actually happens (or
should happen) during your physical examination to find
out if you have fibromyalgia.

Chapter 5

Who Gets Picked to Have Fibromyalgia?

Maybe you're a woman who has fibromyalgia. In addition to you, your sister has it, your daughter has it, and you think that your mother probably has it as well, although she hasn't been diagnosed yet. All the key women in your family seem to have fibromyalgia syndrome (FMS). Not only that, but your brother who served in the Gulf War is also experiencing some symptoms that sound an awful lot like the ones you and your female relatives all share: widespread pain, fatigue, sleep difficulties, and other shared symptoms.

Almost anyone can develop fibromyalgia. But there *are* general patterns among the people who are the most likely to be diagnosed with FMS; for example, women are much more frequently found to have fibromyalgia than are men. (Although men can and do have fibromyalgia.) And adults are more prone to being diagnosed with fibromyalgia than are children.

This chapter covers the types of people most likely to develop fibromyalgia. At the same time, though, it also includes information on men with fibromyalgia who may be even less likely to receive a diagnosis than women. In addition, I discuss a possible explanation for *why* women may suffer from fibromyalgia more than men: In general, women actually experience pain more acutely than men do.

Looking at the Numbers: Who Has FMS?

About 6 million people in the United States and millions more worldwide have fibromyalgia, and the overwhelming majority are adult women who are roughly of childbearing age (about 20–45 years old). Although it's possible for men or for children and adolescents to suffer from the symptoms of fibromyalgia, the majority of people who are diagnosed with FMS are women. Many women diagnosed with fibromyalgia are white women, although women of any race may develop fibromyalgia.

There are several possibilities to consider here. These numbers may exist simply because they're valid, and most of the people who actually do have fibromyalgia really are Caucasian females between these ages. On the other hand, many physicians may not be *looking* for FMS in children, just as they may not be looking for it in males, in women under age 20 or over age 45, in nonwhite women, and so forth. (I cover helping children with fibromyalgia in Chapter 20.) Simply put, if FMS isn't in the doctor's constellation of possibilities, often, he's just not going to find it among his patients.

It's not that he's a bad doctor. Instead, FMS just isn't the first (and maybe not the second, third, fourth, and so on) thing that a physician usually looks for among people who fit into these other groups — even when their symptoms may seem consistent with a diagnosis of fibromyalgia (widespread pain, muscle stiffness, tender points, chronic fatigue, sleep problems, and so on).

As a result, if you don't fit into the basic patterns of people who usually have fibromyalgia, you may want to ask your doctor if you may possibly have this medical problem, even though you're generally regarded as "too young" or "too old" to be considered a candidate — or even though you're a man or an African American or an Asian woman.

Wondering Why Women Suffer More from FMS than Men

If you're a woman, you may have thought that experiencing menstruation and (if you decide to have a child) suffering from labor pains were difficult enough to cope with. Certainly, they can both be painful experiences that are unique to women. (Although, you eventually do gain a child when you have labor pains, which is — for most women — well worth the temporary pain.)

Now, I must also tell you that women are approximately seven times more likely to develop fibromyalgia than men are. Read on for some of the support behind this statistic.

Research has shown that women are significantly more sensitive to painful stimuli than men are, and this pain sensitivity is particularly true with regard to soft tissues and muscles that are examined by physicians. (Soft tissue and muscle pain can stem from damage or defects to the musculoskeletal system, such as strains, tears, or fractures. Rarely, it comes from infections or organic defects or damage, such as heart attack or stroke.) Studies have also revealed that women are often more likely than men to seek out doctors when they feel pain, and they're also more likely than men to complain when they experience pain.

The idea that women are more sensitive to pain than men may possibly blow a hole through the "tough guy" kind of image that some men would like to maintain. Instead of being solidly stoic in the face of pain, they're generally just more impervious to pain than women are. I'm not trying to minimize male pain. It's also real for men, and it also hurts. But it apparently hurts less, in many cases. In fact, some experts believe that women's higher level of pain sensitivity may well be what causes females to become much more at risk for developing fibromyalgia than men.

Or, as the authors of *Muscle Pain: Understanding Its Nature, Diagnosis, and Treatment* (Baltimore, Lippincott, Williams & Wilkins, 2001) put it, "The greater sensitivity of women to painful stimuli may help to explain why there are approximately seven times as many women as men with fibromyalgia." They also added, "It comes as a surprise to many male practitioners that women frequently experience more pain than do men in response to the same stimulus."

It's not that doctors are unappreciative of the pain that women suffer from. Instead, the reality is that many physicians, along with most people in the general public, haven't learned yet about studies indicating greater pain sensitivity among women. But medical school professors like me are working hard to find out why women actually hurt more than men do. And until more studies are performed to determine gender pain differences among men and women with fibromyalgia, the issue remains up in the air.

Considering How FMS Relates to Women's Ages

FMS is most commonly diagnosed in women who are between the ages of 20 and 45. In this section, I give you more information on how age and FMS correlate in women of different ages.

Young women

Young women may find that they're experiencing the onset of their fibromyalgia symptoms, or they may have had FMS for years. (I'm defining *young women* as females who are ages 18 to about 39, after which they can be better defined as women who are in their middle years.) They also may be prone to trying hard to ignore the problem, concentrating instead on the demands of their jobs and their children, and trying to work despite their pain and fatigue.

Putting off acknowledging that you have FMS is a mistake. You're better off if you work on your medical problems when they first develop because you have a good chance of preventing them from getting much worse. You can't stop yourself from aging. But if you know that you have fibromyalgia as a young woman, with the help of your physician, you can work on creating a good plan of exercise, weight loss, and pain control. This plan may help you to shortstop a future that's clouded with much greater pain and more limitations than you currently face.

Middle-aged women

Many women in early middle age (I'm defining *middle age* as 40 to 64 years old) are more likely to experience problems with obesity and the onset of other health problems, such as arthritis. Fibromyalgia and its symptoms may be a burden that's laid on top of other emerging and serious health problems that middle-aged women experience.

FMS doesn't seem to have a link to *perimenopause* (the onset of menopause) or menopause, although studies need to be done to determine if such a connection may exist. However, stress is strongly linked to fibromyalgia, and many women in middle age, especially in their 40's and early 50's, are members of the "sandwich generation," and they're responsible for teenage children as well as care giving for their aging parents. The stress that comes with this difficult role may trigger fibromyalgia in women who are predisposed to the problem.

Older women

No one knows how many older women (and men) may suffer from fibromyalgia, but it seems likely that at least some do. In fact, one isolated study indicated that FMS actually *peaked* at age 70, after which it appeared to drop off in incidence. However, more studies need to be performed on people over age 65 to determine the extent of fibromyalgia among the geriatric population.

The trouble with "women's troubles"

Laurie's had fibromyalgia symptoms her entire life. But they've always been perceived as symptoms that were related to her gender. She says that when she started getting her period, the symptoms were always related to menstruation — because she was going to get her period or because she had her period or even because her period had just finished. Somehow, the pain in her body was always related to the bleeding, according to the doctors.

When she got older, the problem became, "getting older." Laurie suspects that at some point in the future, when she goes through menopause, doctors will say that menopause is causing all her body aches. Laurie says that it's almost like being female is a disease. (If you think that your doctor regards womanhood as a disease like Laurie's doctors did, be sure to read Chapter 7 on dealing with your doctor or finding a new physician.)

One possibility is that older people may have FMS, but they also may have other medical problems that are so severe that they require a great deal of attention, such as a history of stroke, cancer, heart attack, severe osteoarthritis, diabetes, or other ailments. As a result, fibromyalgia may not seem like such a big deal to physicians in comparison to these other, often life-threatening, medical problems. (Although FMS is very painful, it's not a life-threatening condition.) It's also true that sometimes FMS symptoms might be ignored or even diagnosed as "you're just getting older" by some physicians.

FMS and Men: It Isn't Just a Woman Thing

Although the overwhelming majority of people who are diagnosed with fibromyalgia are women, it's possible for a man to have FMS, too. In fact, considering the major difficulty that some women report that they've had to go through in obtaining a diagnosis of fibromyalgia, a man with the same medical problem may have an even harder time receiving an accurate diagnosis of his condition.

Some men with fibromyalgia are military veterans, particularly from the Gulf War. (For more information on this topic, read Chapter 3.) Whether they're veterans or nonveterans, however, the symptoms that men experience are generally the same as the symptoms felt by women, although some men with fibromyalgia report that their fatigue is more troublesome than the pain. Unfortunately, the reality is that insufficient studies have been performed on men who have been diagnosed with fibromyalgia to provide any level of detailed information.

Until that problem is rectified, doctors and others can't know for sure whether fibromyalgia has gender differences, both in terms of the types of symptoms that men experience and in their overall severity.

However, as male patients and their doctors become more aware of the very existence of fibromyalgia, and the reality that it's a problem that men can and do have, the probability of an accurate diagnosis and good treatment will increase.

Tom, 42, says that he had a difficult time obtaining a diagnosis, and it wasn't until he asked his doctor if his problem could be the same thing as Tom's sister (who had been diagnosed with fibromyalgia) that it occurred to the physician to consider fibromyalgia. After the doctor started thinking about FMS as a possibility for Tom's tender points, fatigue, and other symptoms, he said that it seemed very obvious that fibromyalgia was the correct diagnosis for Tom's condition. The possibility just hadn't occurred to him before.

Consequently, men who think that they may have fibromyalgia should ask their doctors about it because some men do suffer from FMS.

Chapter 6

Identifying Diseases Often Confused with Fibromyalgia

*Y*ou may wonder *why* you should care about other medical problems that can be confused with fibromyalgia syndrome (FMS) and why I've devoted an entire chapter to this topic. Self-empowerment is the reason why. If you're diagnosed with one of these other problems but you're not getting better with treatment, you may have fibromyalgia instead. In addition, many people with fibromyalgia also suffer from one or more of the medical conditions described in this chapter.

Yet, sometimes, doctors may diagnose *only* your arthritis or *only* your thyroid disease, for example, and not your fibromyalgia. The reverse is also possible. You may be diagnosed with *only* fibromyalgia when you could also have thyroid disease, arthritis, or another medical problem. Knowing about these other health problems can help you become a better informed health consumer.

I'm starting my discussion with medical problems that can be fibromyalgia imposters (medical problems with symptoms like fibromyalgia, and which may confuse or delay the diagnosis) or fibromyalgia cohabitors (conditions that you may have in addition to fibromyalgia) with chronic fatigue syndrome (CFS). Then I move to other conditions that are also sometimes confused with fibromyalgia.

In addition, I also cover several other conditions that have symptoms similar to fibromyalgia, including Lyme disease, mononucleosis, lower back conditions, reflex sympathetic dystrophy, and multiple chemical sensitivities syndrome.

Understanding the Uncertainty

Lauren's doctor had explained to her that her x-rays, along with her symptoms of pain and muscle stiffness, clearly indicated that she had arthritis. He even pointed out the proof to her, using the x-rays to illustrate where the problems were in her neck and back.

Lauren had been faithfully following her doctor's treatment recommendations of medication and exercise, and she felt *some* better. Yet a lot of the pain was still there and, what was really weird, it even seemed to move around from place to place sometimes. Could arthritis do *that*? Lauren also had trouble sleeping at night. And she was very tired, nearly all the time.

Lauren went back to the doctor and asked him to please reconsider her condition. Could something more than arthritis be at work here? Her physician carefully reviewed Lauren's symptoms, her lab tests, and her medical history and then came to his diagnosis. The doctor told Lauren that she really did have arthritis, as he'd diagnosed her with before — AND she also had fibromyalgia. The pain that moved from place to place, along with her other symptoms of insomnia and fatigue, had tipped him off to the fibromyalgia.

Doctors should easily be able to distinguish fibromyalgia syndrome (FMS) from all other medical conditions, shouldn't they? After all, they're smart, they went to medical school, and they're trained in the scientific method. It should be a piece of cake for them, right? Unfortunately, this viewpoint has several gaping problems.

One problem is that many different symptoms overlap between fibromyalgia and an array of other frequently occurring medical problems. In fact, even trained physicians often initially confuse fibromyalgia with several other medical problems that may be present in their patients, such as chronic fatigue syndrome (CFS), myofascial pain syndrome, arthritis, or thyroid disease.

To muddy the water even further, many people don't have *only* fibromyalgia, but instead, they also have other medical conditions along with the fibromyalgia, just as in Lauren's case. In these circumstances, these other medical problems can easily distract the physician from the diagnosis of fibromyalgia. As a result, you shouldn't be surprised that, sometimes, people may be underdiagnosed — even by good physicians.

Happily, most physicians are becoming increasingly adept at correctly identifying and distinguishing fibromyalgia from other possible medical problems, and they're also getting better at effectively treating their patients who have FMS. But, to be on the safe side, consumers should also have a basic general understanding of the other diseases that can so often become confused with FMS, as well as an understanding of the differences between fibromyalgia and other major medical problems. Such knowledge may also give readers the confidence to ask their doctors more questions, as Lauren did.

Chronic Fatigue Syndrome

Chronic fatigue syndrome (CFS) is a condition that's characterized by severe and long-term fatigue and exhaustion. It's also known as *chronic fatigue/immune dysfunction syndrome,* or CFIDS.

I start with CFS because it's probably the condition that's most frequently confused with fibromyalgia. This confusion results partly from the fact that patients with chronic fatigue syndrome often share many of the same symptoms as people with fibromyalgia. Because of this considerable overlap in symptoms, many researchers actually consider CFS as a special form of fibromyalgia.

Although the two syndromes have many points of intersection, fibromyalgia and chronic fatigue syndrome are actually different illnesses. Researchers have found subtle differences between CFS patients and FMS patients. However, diagnosis can be very difficult when the patient is burdened with symptoms of *both* fibromyalgia and chronic fatigue syndrome — which, unfortunately, can happen sometimes.

About CFS

The prevailing symptom of chronic fatigue syndrome is an extreme and overwhelming long-term exhaustion.

Patients with chronic fatigue syndrome say that this exhaustion goes way beyond the mere tiredness that most people without CFS feel from time to time. People who have CFS say that they feel completely overwhelmed and totally drained of all energy, even when they haven't been doing anything that would normally cause minor fatigue.

With FMS, in contrast, the fatigue that patients feel is usually listed as their second worst problem, or it may be even farther down on their list of most aggravating symptoms. Instead, pain's the paramount complaint for people who have FMS.

CDC guidelines for diagnosing CFS

The *Centers for Disease Control and Prevention* (CDC), the federal agency that provides information and guidance on major diseases and medical conditions, has created guidelines to diagnose chronic fatigue syndrome based on symptoms. These guidelines can be briefly summarized as the following:

✔ The patient has had unexplained fatigue for six months or more. This fatigue isn't caused by physical exertion and doesn't go away or even improve with rest.

✔ The patient's work, educational, social, and personal activities have been affected by this persistent fatigue.

✔ The patient has also experienced four or more of the following symptoms: sore throat, muscle pain, difficulty with concentration or short-term memory, headaches that are unlike headaches experienced in the past, joint pain in more than one joint but without accompanying redness or inflammation, sleep that is not refreshing, and malaise that occurs after physical exertion and lasts for at least 24 hours.

Besides fatigue, many other symptoms are associated with having chronic fatigue syndrome, such as an overall malaise, a hypersensitivity to lights and noise, and chronic headaches in people who never had such frequent headaches prior to their onset of CFS. People with chronic fatigue syndrome may also suffer from other symptoms, such as *hypotension* (low blood pressure), and *syncope* (fainting).

In addition, many patients with CFS are also prone to developing *irritable bowel syndrome* (IBS), which means that they have varying degrees of belly pain with diarrhea or constipation. These problems are also common to people who have fibromyalgia, and thus, physicians may have a hard time determining whether CFS or fibromyalgia is the appropriate diagnosis.

How CFS differs from fibromyalgia

The difficulty in distinguishing CFS from fibromyalgia is sometimes complicated by the fact that, sadly, some people alternate between *both* medical conditions. As a result, the physician may find it hard to diagnose each individual medical problem.

In general, if pain is the main complaint and the patient has other symptoms of fibromyalgia, such as *tender points* (specific areas of the body that are sore, described in more detail in Chapter 8), the medical problem is probably fibromyalgia.

In contrast, if the patient's key complaint is extreme fatigue, followed by other symptoms, such as pain and sleep difficulties, CFS is more likely to be diagnosed as the prevailing problem.

Because these two syndromes are more frequently confused than the other medical problems that I discuss in this chapter, I provide you a chart (Table 6-1) that compares the key symptoms of fibromyalgia and of chronic fatigue syndrome.

Table 6-1	Comparing Chronic Fatigue Syndrome (CFS) to Fibromyalgia	
Symptom/Finding	*Fibromyalgia*	*Chronic Fatigue Syndrome*
Pain	Primary symptom	Secondary symptom
Fatigue	Secondary symptom	Primary symptom
High spinal fluid levels of Substance P	Yes	No
Physical brain changes	No	Maybe (cortical white matter lesions)
Abnormal growth hormone levels	Yes, in some patients	No
Problems with concentration	Yes	Yes
Chronic or frequent sore throat	No	Yes
Problems with short-term memory	Yes	Yes
Tender lymph nodes	No	Yes
Chronic low-grade fever	No	Yes

Treating CFS

Although chronic fatigue syndrome currently has no cure, the condition eventually does appear to improve in most people — but how long it takes to feel better varies from person to person. In the meantime, physicians can treat CFS patients by using medications such as nonsteroidal anti-inflammatory drugs and low doses of antidepressants. (Read more about medications in Chapters 9 and 10.) Some physicians also place their patients with CFS on antiviral regimens or on antibiotics.

For further information and for the latest findings on chronic fatigue syndrome and related issues, contact the national charitable group, the CFIDS Association of America, P.O. Box 220398, Charlotte, NC 28222-0398; phone 800-442-3437 or 704-365-2343 (resource line); Web site www.cfids.org.

Considering cortisol

Could cortisol (a hormone released by the adrenal glands that helps to control blood pressure, blood sugar, and other major body functions) be the key to both the cause of chronic fatigue syndrome and its solution? Researchers who performed a study of 32 CFS patients reported on their findings in the British medical journal *Lancet* in 1999. The researchers found that about one-third of their subjects significantly improved upon taking low doses of oral hydrocortisone, a synthetically made form of cortisol (5 or 10 milligrams per day), and subsequently felt much more energetic.

The researchers hypothesized that *hypocortisolism*, or a below-normal rate of the cortisol hormone produced by the adrenal glands, may have been responsible for the fatigue experienced by the patients. However, hydrocortisone is an experimental treatment, and further studies need to be done before hydrocortisone can be considered as an acceptable treatment for patients who have chronic fatigue syndrome.

Looking at lifestyle changes

Doctors may also give patients with CFS lifestyle change recommendations, such as advice on exercising and, if needed, weight loss as well. ***Note:*** Because people with CFS are very easily overtired, they should exercise at a slow rate.

Walking and mild aerobic exercises are usually best for individuals with chronic fatigue syndrome. In addition to physical activity, the individual may also frequently benefit from psychological counseling because depression or anxiety often accompanies CFS.

Myofascial Pain Syndrome

Another condition that often may be confused with fibromyalgia is *myofascial pain syndrome* (MFS). This syndrome is primarily characterized by *regional pain*, or pain that's confined to one particular area. This type of pain differs from the more widespread pain that's so characteristic of patients with fibromyalgia. In addition, the doctor can also identify the painful areas when he probes them, because they feel ropey, like knotted ropes or nodular to the touch.

Experts say that many cases of MFS have gone undiagnosed, despite the severity of the case. Yet this medical problem is usually treatable with medications and other therapies.

About myofascial pain syndrome

MFS may be caused or worsened by mechanical stress or strain on the muscles, such as from heavy lifting, a physically traumatizing event, or by overstressing the muscles of the body in some other manner. Whatever caused the muscle groups to become stressed, they stay that way and cause pain.

MFS occurs about equally among women and men, which is in sharp contrast to patients with fibromyalgia — a medical problem that's dominated by female patients. (Not that women _want_ to be the FMS leaders. It just happens to work out that way.)

Pain that's caused by MFS occurs most commonly in the head, shoulders, or the lower back (and usually not in all those places, as is common with fibromyalgia). Pain from neck muscles can radiate into the skull, although any muscles anywhere in the body can develop trigger points.

Trigger points are areas of pain that are characteristic of myofascial pain syndrome. A trigger point is a ropey or nodular muscle area that causes pain and that can be felt in one or more areas of the body by the doctor when he or she probes the painful area. They're very different from the _tender points_ of fibromyalgia, which are located in many different parts of the body and can't be felt by the doctor.

With fibromyalgia, your painful areas, or tender points, are very sore to the touch for you, but the physician doesn't usually feel anything during your physical examination, even when directly probing the areas that cause you pain. In fact, the person with FMS feels basically the same to him as another person who does not have FMS, even in the sore areas. The pain is really there when you have fibromyalgia, but it's just not related to specific muscle abnormalities.

Several other key features characterize myofascial pain syndrome. They are:

- ✔ **Regional pain, rather than the widespread pain found in fibromyalgia.** The person with FMS may feel pain in her neck, shoulders, upper back, lower back, in other sites, or in all these areas. The pain may also alternate from one site to another. With myofascial syndrome, the pain takes up permanent residence in one or several different hurtful places, and it stays there for a long time.

- ✔ **A limited mobility of motion.** With myofascial pain syndrome, you may have local pain with movements. With FMS, on the other hand, moving around a lot may hurt, but the pain is usually scattered and widespread.

- ✔ **A good response to trigger-point injections of medication.** With FMS, the patient usually doesn't get similar pain relief from trigger point injections. Besides, how many trigger-point injections can you get in one sitting anyway? (See the section, "Treating myofascial pain syndrome," later in this chapter for details on trigger-point injections.)

How myofascial pain syndrome differs from FMS

If you read somewhere else or someone tells you that myofascial pain syndrome and fibromyalgia are really the same condition, remember what I'm telling you here: They're not. Although FMS and myofascial syndrome do have many overlapping features and you can actually have *both* medical conditions at the same time, the reality is that they're two very different medical problems.

Emotional problems, such as depression and anxiety, occur more frequently among people with fibromyalgia than among people who have MFS. This doesn't mean that patients with MFS are never depressed or anxious. It just means that they're less likely to have these emotional problems than are people with fibromyalgia.

Another difference is that myofascial pain is usually more localized than the pain from fibromyalgia, which is widespread.

Even though myofascial syndrome is different from fibromyalgia, it does share the common denominator of pain. In addition, many people with MFS also have problems with fatigue and sleep difficulties. However, the *fibro fog,* or major difficulty with concentration, that's characteristic of many people who have fibromyalgia is less frequently found among patients with MFS.

Treating myofascial pain syndrome

Studies indicate that day laborers regularly performing physically demanding manual work are much less prone to developing trigger points than are individuals who are basically sedentary and then suddenly engage in physically demanding tasks. As a result, although exercise and physical activity are generally good for most people, people who are out of shape and who have MFS need to build up slowly from a sedentary level to a more active level. In fact, this policy is good for sedentary people even if they don't have MFS. Build up slowly and safely.

Because specific and identifiable trigger points can be found in myofascial pain syndrome, the condition may be treated with special *trigger-point injections* of medication, inserted directly into the painful areas. (And yes, these injections can hurt at first, but the pain dissipates quickly, and the relief moves in. Most patients consider the relief well worth any temporary discomfort.)

Patients with MFS may also gain good relief with a variety of medications, such as muscle relaxants, nonsteroidal anti-inflammatory medications, and painkilling drugs. These medications are discussed in Chapters 9 and 10.

Biofeedback therapy may also be helpful to patients with myofascial pain syndrome, in that it can help very tense patients receive training in how to relax their overstressed muscles that are causing them such pain. Relaxation therapy may help as well. (Read more about these therapies in Chapter 13.)

Arthritis

Some people with fibromyalgia may be told that they have arthritis — and the doctor may be right because arthritis is very commonly associated with FMS. Very generally, arthritis is a disease of the joints and the surrounding tissues. Arthritis actually has many different forms, but two primary types are the arthritis leaders, in terms of their incidence among people in the general population. These two types are *osteoarthritis* and *rheumatoid arthritis*.

Physicians may sometimes assume that patients have one of these forms of arthritis, particularly osteoarthritis (because it's so common), when the primary problem may be fibromyalgia instead. Also, patients may actually have osteoarthritis along with fibromyalgia, or they may have both rheumatoid arthritis and fibromyalgia.

About arthritis

The long-term damage that's caused by osteoarthritis (and sometimes by rheumatoid arthritis as well) can be so severe that the affected person will eventually require joint replacements, usually of the knee or the hip joints. If a person is diagnosed with a severe case of osteoarthritis or rheumatoid arthritis, the physician may want to concentrate primarily on this medical problem because of its potentially damaging effects. As a result, he or she may altogether miss the diagnosis of a coexisting problem with fibromyalgia.

The key characteristics of arthritis are pain and inflammation, and clinical tests, such as x-rays, blood tests, or the doctor's visual observation of apparent swelling and damage of a patient's joint, usually show some abnormalities. In general, people with fibromyalgia and no arthritis have normal x-rays and normal blood test results, and their friends and relatives drive them crazy by telling them that they look "just fine."

Boning up on osteoarthritis

Osteoarthritis is the most prominent form of arthritis. It's a disease in which the cartilage and the bones steadily degenerate, often causing moderate to severe pain in the joints that usually worsens as the person ages.

Osteoarthritis is a degenerative "wear and tear" disease of the bones. Although people often think of older people when they think of osteoarthritis, you don't have to be a senior citizen to be diagnosed with osteoarthritis; middle-aged or even younger individuals may also be diagnosed with osteoarthritis.

As people with osteoarthritis age, their condition usually worsens. Their pain increases, and their x-rays usually show an increased deterioration compared to past x-rays. In fact, the damage can become quite severe, although treatment can often delay the progression of this disease. Given a choice between fibromyalgia and arthritis (if that were possible!), you may think twice before choosing arthritis.

Regarding rheumatoid arthritis

The other common form of arthritis is *rheumatoid arthritis*, an inflammatory form of arthritis that causes swelling, stiffness, and the eventual deformity and destruction of the joints.

Rheumatoid arthritis (RA) is an *autoimmune disorder*, or a disorder in which the person's immune system mistakenly attacks its own tissues as if they were foreign invaders that must be attacked, like a virus or bacteria. Rheumatoid arthritis causes pain, inflammation, and damage to the joints. In many people, RA becomes progressively worse with aging.

Severe morning stiffness is a common symptom of RA, as is debilitating pain in the joints. Rheumatoid arthritis usually has an onset in patients between the ages of 20 and 45, although it can develop earlier or later in a person's life. Women have about four times the risk of developing rheumatoid arthritis as men do, which is related to the fact that in general, women are more likely to experience autoimmune disorders than men.

Laboratory tests can usually (about 60 percent of the time) detect particular blood factors that are indicators for the presence or at least the likelihood of rheumatoid arthritis. In addition, the damage to the person's joints, which may be swollen and distorted, may be clearly visible to the physician as well as the lay person.

In the early stages of the condition, however, the diagnosis of arthritis may be missed, particularly if the patient was previously diagnosed with fibromyalgia. And the reverse is true: If the patient was previously diagnosed with arthritis, the diagnosis of fibromyalgia may be missed.

How arthritis differs from fibromyalgia

How can either form of arthritis possibly be confused with fibromyalgia? This confusion can occur in two primary cases. First, the osteoarthritis or rheumatoid arthritis may be an early case, and damage is not yet detectable in lab work or x-rays.

In the early stages of arthritis, the disease causes pain, muscle stiffness, overall achiness, and fatigue. Patients may also experience symptoms of depression and anxiety, as they also do with fibromyalgia. The doctor may assume that if the patient's symptoms sound like arthritis, it *must* be arthritis.

Another reason for missing the diagnosis of FMS is that many people with fibromyalgia actually do have arthritis as well because arthritis is a very common medical problem. As a result, the diagnosis of arthritis may be correctly flagged by the physician, but the identification of fibromyalgia as a major player in the patient's pain and other symptoms may be altogether missed.

What if a person has *only* fibromyalgia? Can she be misdiagnosed with arthritis? Yes, this can happen when the mistaken diagnosis is osteoarthritis, primarily because osteoarthritis is so commonly found. Even if no extensive damage can be found in x-rays, physicians may still assume that the person is suffering from a "touch" of arthritis, which usually means that the patient has indications of early osteoarthritis. But the correct diagnosis may be fibromyalgia instead.

Treating arthritis

If you're diagnosed with arthritis, your doctor should be able to help you improve how you feel. However, keep in mind that, as with fibromyalgia, arthritis is a chronic disease, and no magic pills are out there that can eradicate it forever.

Whether you have rheumatoid arthritis or osteoarthritis, the key elements of help for both forms of arthritis are medication, exercises to improve your stiffness and your range of motion, and basic lifestyle changes, such as weight loss (when needed) and a nutritious diet. Physical therapy may also provide some relief.

Medicating arthritis

People with osteoarthritis generally need medications in a class known as *nonsteroidal anti-inflammatory drugs*, or NSAIDs. These medications are taken to reduce pain that stems from inflammation. As the name stipulates, they aren't steroid drugs. NSAIDs are available in both over-the-counter and prescribed strengths. Their primary side effect is to cause stomach upset, and their continued use may cause stomach ulcers.

Rheumatoid arthritis is treated with a variety of medications. Although most anti-inflammatory drugs and mild painkillers may provide pain relief to patients with rheumatoid arthritis, most patients will also need to receive drugs in the disease-modifying antirheumatic (DMARD) class, such as methotrexate sulfasalazine, hydroxychloroquine, or intramuscular gold injections.

Doctors may suggest prescribing a DMARD drug early in the course of the disease because these drugs can prevent serious joint damage.

Newer drugs for rheumatoid arthritis include Enbrel (generic name: etanercept) and Remicade (generic name: inflixamab), both drugs that work to block inflammation. Patients may also be given drugs in the *COX-2 inhibitor class* to block inflammation and pain, such as Celebrex (generic name: celecoxib) and Vioxx (generic name: rofecoxib).

Considering other needed treatments

The patient with rheumatoid arthritis may also need to "rest" a joint, with the use of splints or braces. Some patients in the later stages of rheumatoid arthritis may be so impaired that they may require a walker in order to move about.

People with arthritis can often gain considerable benefit from cold or heat therapy or from massage therapy (as described in Chapter 11), as well as from relaxation therapy, (covered in Chapter 13). Aquatic exercises and swimming may also improve their problems with physical mobility and pain. (Read more about how exercise can help your fibromyalgia symptoms in Chapter 15.) Low doses of antidepressants, as described in Chapter 10, may also help decrease pain and may work to improve sleep among those with sleep problems.

These are all therapies, which, coincidentally, also benefit people with FMS. As a result, if you happen to have the dubious honor of having both arthritis and fibromyalgia, such therapies can help you to improve both conditions.

Thyroid Disease

Now, arthritis and fibromyalgia seem to go together quite well. But how could anyone possibly confuse thyroid disease with fibromyalgia? One is an endocrine disorder, and the other is a musculoskeletal problem — two seemingly disparate medical issues.

The key reason why thyroid disease can be easily confused with fibromyalgia is that *hypothyroidism*, or low thyroid function, leads to fatigue and may also cause painful and aching muscles and even widespread pain — the same symptoms that are experienced by most people with fibromyalgia. Hypothyroidism is very common, and it often goes undetected. Yet testing for low thyroid isn't difficult.

If you think that you may have fibromyalgia, you should ask your doctor for a thyroid function blood test to rule out an underactive thyroid gland. If you do have an underactive thyroid, a small thyroid pill, taken once a day, can usually rectify the problem.

About hypothyroidism (low thyroid)

The thyroid gland is an important organ located in your neck. It produces thyroid hormone, a hormone needed for survival. This hormone controls a person's basic energy level and affects many aspects of the body, such as blood pressure, heart rate, and even fertility and mood states. People need thyroid hormone to live, whether from their own thyroid gland or from thyroid supplement medications that they take.

Sometimes, people develop thyroid problems that cause low or high levels of thyroid hormone to circulate in the body, and this malfunction directly affects the individual. Thyroid disease is almost always treatable, although people with thyroid problems should consult with an *endocrinologist,* a physician who specializes in endocrine diseases like thyroid disorders.

If a person really has a problem with thyroid disease that doctors may confuse with fibromyalgia, it's almost always hypothyroidism. This diagnostic confusion can come from the fact that the symptoms that are more commonly associated with low levels of thyroid, such as low energy, fatigue, and body aches and pains, are also symptoms of fibromyalgia.

The specific screening test for thyroid disorders is called a test for *thyroid-stimulating hormone*, or TSH. If your thyroid gland isn't producing enough thyroid hormone to meet your needs, your pituitary gland will react and raise the level of TSH in your blood. This TSH level is what the test is looking for.

A repeat TSH test is usually done to confirm hypothyroidism before medication is started. There are other thyroid tests, but most doctors consider the TSH to be the "gold standard" of thyroid tests.

If you do have a thyroid disease, you'll need periodic testing of your blood to ensure that the medication is at the right level.

Treating thyroid disease

Hypothyroidism is readily treatable by experienced physicians. Thyroid disease is best treated by *endocrinologists*, or physicians who are experts in treating thyroid diseases and other medical problems that are related to the endocrine system.

Hypothyroidism is treated with prescribed synthetic or natural thyroid hormone, which is available at virtually any pharmacy. The medication is usually taken once daily, and it is best taken on an empty stomach to obtain full potency.

When thyroid disease is first diagnosed and treatment has begun, the TSH is usually repeated several times the first year of treatment, to ensure that the person doesn't need a higher or a lower dosage. After apparent stabilization, the TSH testing may be limited to an annual test, if the doctor decides that's sufficient. Pregnancy or menopause may require a change in the dosage of the drug.

The Other Suspects

In addition to the diseases and medical conditions that I discuss earlier in this chapter, the specific medical problem that causes pain, fatigue, and other symptoms that are characteristic of fibromyalgia may actually be caused by yet another underlying disease or condition.

There are too many possibilities to name them all here, but several are worth discussing, including Lyme disease, reflex sympathetic dystrophy, various medical conditions that cause back pain, and infectious mononucleosis.

Being ticked off by Lyme disease

Lyme disease is an infection caused by an organism with a tongue twister name: *Borrelia burgdorferi*. It's spread by tiny, dot-like ticks that typically feed off animals but aren't opposed to a human treat. If they latch on to you, you could get the disease.

Lyme disease was originally thought to be confined only to the northeast part of the United States and was first identified in Lyme, Connecticut. However, subsequent incidences of Lyme disease were identified in nearly every state throughout the country, as faraway from Connecticut as California. In addition, Lyme disease has also been identified in European countries, such as France, Germany, and Switzerland, and in Australia and other countries around the world.

Lyme disease can be cured if treated early on, but if the disease goes undiagnosed for months or longer, then it usually becomes a chronic illness.

You don't have to have an up-close and personal encounter with an animal in the forest in order to be afflicted by Lyme disease. You can become a tick's host if you go out walking in deep grass or if you interact a lot with your pets who go outside. What if you never saw any ticks on your body? Doesn't that mean that you're safe from Lyme disease? Sorry, but it doesn't. Experts say that most patients who have tested positive for Lyme never recall seeing a tick on themselves.

Some of the symptoms of Lyme disease may resemble those of fibromyalgia, such as widespread joint pain, fatigue, difficulty concentrating, and so forth. Flu-like symptoms occur in the first stage of Lyme disease, and a characteristic rash typically occurs. The symptoms generally escalate several weeks or even months later to musculoskeletal pain, arthritis, and swelling. These symptoms may be clinically confused with fibromyalgia or with osteoarthritis.

As with all the other medical problems that are described in this chapter, patients can have both FMS and Lyme disease. However, unlike with rheumatoid arthritis or fibromyalgia, the arthritis of Lyme disease is usually limited to one joint, most often the knee, and it is difficult to overlook.

One laboratory indicator of possible Lyme disease is an elevated *erythrocyte sedimentation rate* (ESR, also called the "sed rate" by doctors), an indicator of inflammation, anemia, and increased white blood cell count. Doctors may suspect that Lyme disease is present, based on your symptoms and the ESR, but the illness can really only be confirmed with further testing that the doctor orders.

In most cases, doctors order a blood test called a *Lyme titer*, which is a special test that checks for Lyme disease. If this test turns out to be positive, other confirming tests are also ordered. The Lyme titer does have some false negatives, especially if the person has just contracted the disease, but these false negatives aren't common.

Making sure that people actually have Lyme disease before any treatment is initiated is important because the treatment can be long and costly, particularly when the disease is identified in the late stages. In the early stages, patients may be treated with oral antibiotics for about two to three weeks. However, if the disease has progressed to a later stage, patients must take the antibiotics intravenously for at least several weeks — possibly for several months.

These drugs can be administered to you in your home with the help of trained medical people, or you may be able to find out how to administer them yourself, with the help of another person. The antibiotics that are used are very strong and may lead to other side effects, such as an overgrowth of yeast or gastrointestinal side effects.

Evaluating other possibilities

Your doctor may consider a variety of other ailments when trying to make a diagnosis when pain is present. Ailments that cause low back pain are one possibility. Other far less common medical problems are reflex sympathetic dystrophy, multiple chemical sensitivities syndrome, and mononucleosis.

Low back pain

The majority of all adults experience pain in their lower backs at some time in their lives. If the pain is chronic, it may indicate some minor or moderate damage to the spine. The underlying problem causing your symptoms may also be arthritis. Or, it could be disk problem, infection, or something else. The causes of low back pain are numerous.

Low back pain may also indicate fibromyalgia, particularly if other symptoms are present, such as pain in other parts of the body, fatigue, and sleep difficulties.

When patients complain primarily of low back pain, doctors try to determine if a recent injury, such as a fall or car crash, occurred. If not, they seek to determine other possible causes, such as a kidney infection, bladder infection, or some other internal problem.

Physicians usually order a complete blood count and a variety of other blood tests, as well as a urinalysis, to detect bacteria or blood, in case the underlying problem is a bladder infection or a urinary tract infection. They may also order spinal x-rays to help them determine if the pain comes from damage to the spinal cord or from arthritis.

If the low back pain has continued without any relief for weeks or months and the physician suspects a serious problem (or wants to rule one out), he may order a *magnetic resonance imaging (MRI)* scan. An MRI is an expensive special test that is noninvasive and provides many details of bones, muscles, tissues, and internal organs. If the patient has normal laboratory tests, normal x-rays, and, if ordered, a normal MRI, the problem may be fibromyalgia.

Reflex sympathetic dystrophy

Another medical condition that may be confused with fibromyalgia is *reflex sympathetic dystrophy* (RSD), which is also known as *complex regional pain syndrome*. This illness is a serious and painful condition that's most frequently found in the patient's arms or legs. This medical problem may result from muscles that are damaged at the microscopic level or by an unexplained hypersensitivity of the nerve endings found in the painful area. In addition, the skin of the painful area usually appears shiny to both medical doctors and laypersons. The affected area may also feel cool compared to the other parts of the body.

Reflex sympathetic dystrophy is often so painful that the person tries to avoid moving the affected limb altogether. Unfortunately, this attempt to never move the arm or leg ultimately worsens the pain further.

This medical problem is primarily treated with sedatives, anticonvulsants, and various forms of painkilling medications. Antidepressants may also be helpful for patients to help them sleep. Some patients need anti-anxiety drugs as well.

Rest is usually also recommended. In addition, RSD is also treated with physical therapy, massage, and exercises. Sometimes, *transcutaneous electrical nerve stimulation (TENS),* a treatment of painless electrical impulses applied to the affected areas, offers some relief to the person with reflex sympathetic dystrophy.

Multiple chemical sensitivities syndrome

A very controversial diagnosis, *multiple chemical sensitivities syndrome* (MCSS), means that the patient has seemingly become extremely sensitive to many different substances that have never bothered him or her before, such as numerous odors, foods, and other common items that are found in most environments.

Items like perfumes, household detergents, and cigarette smoke can induce severe symptoms, such as migraine headaches, insomnia, joint pain, and mental confusion. These are, coincidentally, also symptoms that can occur in a person who has fibromyalgia.

This syndrome is sometimes confused with the "boy in the bubble" situation, a very unique situation in which a child had virtually no immune system and had to live confined in a special bacteria-free environment because any germs would've killed him. But people with MCSS still have working immune systems, even though it may seem to them that everything bothers them and causes them to have symptoms.

Narrowing down the specific causes of what's aggravating their fatigue and pain and other symptoms can be a major challenge for both the patient and the doctor. No blood tests or other laboratory screening measures that currently exist can screen for multiple chemical sensitivities syndrome; consequently, this diagnosis is generally made based on the observations of the physician — and only long after all other possible causes are completely ruled out.

Mononucleosis

Can adults contact infectious *mononucleosis,* a virus that was once known as the "kissing disease?" Yes, people of any age can contract mononucleosis, the infection obtained through the Epstein-Barr virus.

The basic symptoms of *mono* are fatigue and flu-like aches and pains, which are symptoms also found in fibromyalgia. However, unlike fibromyalgia, the person with mononucleosis often has a sore throat and swollen glands. Fortunately, mononucleosis does eventually go away, with rest and treatment. (Although people can contract mononucleosis more than once.)

The illness is easily screened for with a blood test. If the test is negative, the person usually doesn't have mononucleosis. If the physician doesn't order the Epstein-Barr virus blood test to rule out this illness (because of managed care constraints or for some other reason), he may go ahead and assume that mononucleosis is present, and he may not suspect that the patient really has fibromyalgia.

If the patient doesn't improve with time, the doctor should consider fibromyalgia or other medical problems.

Chapter 7

Working with a Good Fibromyalgia Doc: You Need a True Believer

*L*inda saw an internist, a family practitioner, and two rheumatologists before she was finally diagnosed with fibromyalgia. Sam says that he saw five different doctors. He's forgotten what all their specialties were, but it wasn't until he saw a pain management expert that he was finally diagnosed with fibromyalgia. Amy was lucky compared to most people who are ultimately diagnosed with fibromyalgia syndrome (FMS): She hit the jackpot on her second try and was diagnosed with fibromyalgia about eight months after the first symptoms hit her hard.

Linda, Sam, and Amy all really needed a good doctor, but connecting with one took considerable time. In fact, some people with fibromyalgia are probably never diagnosed or are misdiagnosed for years. Why does this happen? One reason is that a lot of doctors don't understand fibromyalgia. Yet you really need a good, caring, and knowledgeable doctor to help you cope with the pain, fatigue, and other troubling symptoms that fibromyalgia causes.

This chapter is about working with your primary care physician, and it's also about finding another doctor or locating a specialist if you need one. A key point to keep in mind is that you need a doctor who's familiar with the diagnosis and treatment of musculoskeletal pain syndromes like FMS. Many primary care physicians have experience with FMS, but, sometimes, a specialist like a rheumatologist or a neurologist is required to make the diagnosis.

Working with Your Primary Care Doctor

In many cases, your "regular" physician can readily diagnose and treat your fibromyalgia, and you won't need to see any other doctors to receive their specialty knowledge or instructions. Over the last several years, most physicians have begun to realize and accept that FMS is a valid diagnosis. (Although, as mentioned, some skeptical doctors and also some total nonbelievers are still out there.)

Sometimes, however, your primary care doctor may need to look up a few things about fibromyalgia, and he or she may also want to consult with colleagues for their opinions. If so, that's understandable and okay. You may also need a referral to see a specialist, such as a rheumatologist or another type of physician who has more expertise in treating FMS than your primary care doctor possesses.

Happily seeing your doctor who knows about FMS

Ideally, your doctor already knows about fibromyalgia and is treating other patients who have FMS and seeing some improvements in them. I'll call this physician "Doctor Wonderful." Doctor W. is also aware of the many other ailments that are often associated with FMS. (Read Chapter 2 for a complete discussion of the other medical problems that often accompany fibromyalgia.)

In addition to this basic knowledge about fibromyalgia, Doctor W. is also aware of the medications and treatments that usually work best for people with fibromyalgia. (Check out Chapters 9 and 10 for info on FMS-related medications and Chapter 11 for hands-on treatment options.) At the same time, Doctor W. is careful to avoid taking a one-size-fits-all approach because FMS symptoms vary from person to person. Dr. Wonderful is also open to new ideas regarding treatment while retaining a healthy skepticism about new treatments. (I discuss alternative remedies and treatments in Chapter 12.) You're consulting with Dr. W. not only for medical expertise but also for good judgment.

Coping with a doc who's inexperienced but willing to learn

Unfortunately, finding out that your doctor has little experience with FMS is a common problem. Your primary care physician is great for just about everything that ails you. But for some reason, fibromyalgia has him or her thrown for a loop. If your doctor isn't Doctor Wonderful, hopefully he or she is Doctor Good Enough rather than Doctor Awful. Doctor Good Enough may work well for you, if he or she is open-minded, caring, and willing to listen and learn. Check out Table 7-1 for a description of Doctor Good Enough, along with info on how to spot Dr. Wonderful and Dr. Awful as well.

Table 7-1	Comparing Doctors' Approaches to FMS	
Dr. Wonderful	*Dr. Good Enough*	*Dr. Awful*
Knows what fibromyalgia is.	Willing to learn about FMS.	Thinks that FMS is nonsense.
Open-minded about treatment.	Open-minded about treatment.	Resistant to new ideas.
Will help you find a specialist if you need one.	Willing to consider a specialist.	You want a specialist? Go see a psychiatrist.
Sympathetic and caring.	Friendly or neutral.	Disparaging and nasty.
Not a sexist.	Not a sexist.	If you're a woman, the problem always stems from menstruation, pregnancy, or menopause. If you're a man, only women can possibly get fibromyalgia.

Calling Doctor Awful, Doctor Awful

Is every doctor like Dr. Wonderful (or even Doctor Good Enough)? Sadly, the answer is *no.* Therefore, I must introduce you to Doctor Awful. Doctor Awful is the kind of person who doesn't know much about FMS and won't take the time necessary to get to know you and treat your symptoms.

Some doctors continue to see FMS as a nebulous medical problem. Those doctors haven't caught up on the latest scientific data about fibromyalgia. Because they can't see a specific clinical abnormality or result on a lab test or an x-ray, or in some other quantifiable test, they may have trouble making the diagnosis of FMS. They may send off people who suffer from symptoms of chronic pain and fatigue (but who have normal lab results) for psychological counseling only, and they won't prescribe the important comprehensive therapy that's necessary to treat FMS.

Such doctors may assume that the true problem is merely depression and may decide to treat the patients themselves, placing them on moderate to high doses of antidepressants. These doses may have no effect on your fibromyalgia, and they may also cause side effects you don't need, such as excessive sedation and other problems. Actually, low doses of some antidepressants may help alleviate some problems of fibromyalgia, such as pain and sleep difficulties. But in most cases, special medications are needed for moderate to severe pain.

Janet is a physician who suffers from fibromyalgia, and she was diagnosed about a year ago. She says that when she went to medical school, she was taught that fibromyalgia was a problem of neurotic women who constantly felt like they had the flu. Janet isn't surprised, although she's still dismayed, that some people with symptoms of fibromyalgia are sent to mental health professionals to be treated when their primary care doctors receive laboratory reports that are all marked "within the normal range."

Janet is right. Patients need to stand up and speak out that musculoskeletal pain can be a very real problem, and it isn't something you invent to get attention or make people feel sorry for you. FMS sufferers know that they can get attention plenty of other ways, and they also know that most people do *not* feel sorry for those with FMS. Neither Janet nor the overwhelming majority of the other estimated 6 million people with fibromyalgia are malingerers or hypochondriacs.

Looking Elsewhere for a Doctor: How to Know if It's Time

If you've tried to work with your doctor and you feel like you're just not getting anywhere, and if your pain, fatigue, and other symptoms continue to be moderate to severe or are getting worse, you may want to consider working with another physician. It may be the only way for you to get the help that you need.

Every person must make his or her own individual decision about when to seek another medical opinion. But here are some basic points for you to keep in mind before you decide to switch to another doctor or even consult with another physician:

> ✔ **Have you given the doctor enough time to evaluate you and treat you?**
> For example, if you saw the doctor just last week and told him about your problem for the first time, and now you're angry because the first medication didn't work, now's probably too soon to give up on the doctor. In most cases, you should give your physician more time to help you resolve your problem. However, if you've been working with this doctor for months and you don't feel any better at all, it may be time for a change.

✔ **Do you feel that the doctor is taking your problems seriously?** If the doctor hasn't paid enough attention to your symptoms (or you) or has told you that all you need to do is lose weight, exercise, cheer up, or some other simplistic answer, you probably need to think about finding another doctor. These solutions may help you, but they rarely work alone. Instead, most people with fibromyalgia need medications and other treatments.

✔ **Are your doctor's recommendations making you feel *worse* instead of better or about the same?** If the doctor prescribes medications or treatments that exacerbate your condition, you may actually end up feeling worse than you did before. For example, if the doctor recommends vigorous physical therapy and exercise, you need to tell her if this worsens your pain. People with FMS are very pain sensitive, and consequently, they need to exercise at a slower and less intense pace than others who don't have fibromyalgia.

Sometimes, sheer persistence may be needed before you find a doctor who can diagnose and treat your fibromyalgia, although, hopefully, most readers won't have as much trouble as Joan did. Because of severe stiffness in her neck and shoulders, which seemed to appear around the time she was diagnosed with a strep throat, Joan asked her internist for help, but he could find nothing wrong.

Joan changed doctors many times because she felt that they weren't taking her medical problem seriously. In fact, she says that she saw 22 doctors over 18 months until, at long last, she found a rheumatologist who diagnosed her with FMS and treated her. Joan says that the other doctors had told her that her condition was caused by the four pregnancies she'd had and by the onset of menopause. She says that she was angry that the doctors didn't listen to her or believe her, but she's found a good doctor now. Joan is glad that she didn't decide to just settle for one of the other doctors.

Considering Types of Specialists

If your primary care doctor can't or won't treat fibromyalgia or wants you to seek the help or a specialist, not to worry! A variety of specialists treat people with fibromyalgia. Most prominently at the forefront of FMS treatment are rheumatologists, who probably have the most knowledge and information about the syndrome. (However, do *not* assume that all rheumatologists are automatically up to date on fibromyalgia. They're not.)

Neurologists also treat fibromyalgia, as do some doctors among all the specialties who consider themselves to be "pain management specialists." Of course, internists and family practitioners treat FMS, too, but they're generally not regarded as specialists. *Physiatrists* (not psychiatrists, even though the spelling looks very close!), or "sports medicine doctors," also treat ailments like fibromyalgia.

The Fibromyalgia Network is an organization and a source that recommends to callers physicians nationwide who treat fibromyalgia. Contact them at P.O. Box 31750, Tucson, AZ 85751, or call them at their toll-free number: 800-853-2929. (They also have a great newsletter that you can pay to subscribe to.)

Regarding rheumatologists

A *rheumatologist* is an internist (a person who specializes in diseases of the internal system) who further specializes into treating arthritis and diseases of the joints, muscles, and soft tissues. Most rheumatologists are knowledgeable about fibromyalgia. As a result, they should be able to diagnose and treat you effectively with recommended treatments and medications. They should also be able to give you good advice on lifestyle changes that are tailored to your personal needs and that can make you feel better.

Nerving up about neurologists

Neurologists are doctors who specialize in diseases of the brain and nervous system. Because most people with fibromyalgia suffer from severe pain, at some point in their search for a diagnosis, many patients do eventually consult with a neurologist. Many, but not all, neurologists are familiar with fibromyalgia and how it should be diagnosed and treated. Because neurologists are interested in the brain and spinal cord, they're usually aware of problems with pain and the available array of medications to treat pain — as well as with other therapies and lifestyle changes that could help you.

Considering pain management experts

Some doctors specialize in treating all forms of pain and start their own "pain management clinics." Often, these doctors are neurologists or anesthesiologists, although doctors of any specialty may start their own "pain clinic."

Pain management doctors may specialize in certain types of pain, such as the severe pain of cancer or other medical problems that are far more readily diagnosed than fibromyalgia. A pain management clinic may or may not treat a person who has fibromyalgia — the situation varies. Some clinics have told patients that fibromyalgia is "too hard" for them to treat, and they won't accept them as patients. Others have helped FMS patients a great deal.

Pondering other physician specialists

A *physiatrist* is a type of doctor who's familiar with the pros and cons of exercise and physical therapy and who treats injuries that can stem from sports accidents. Sometimes, fibromyalgia results from a physical trauma, such as an athletic accident or a car crash, and physiatrists can help people work on their own rehabilitation.

Doctors who are *orthopedic surgeons* also sometimes treat fibromyalgia. They're knowledgeable about broken bones, sprained ligaments, and muscle injuries, and they can help you create a program of recovery. Of course, whatever specialty the doctor has trained in, he or she needs to be aware of the problems associated with fibromyalgia in particular.

Finding a Good Specialist (Or New Primary Care Doctor)

If you decide that you want to consult with a specialist, where do you start in your search for a smart and knowledgeable doctor who can help you alleviate at least some of the pain and strain of fibromyalgia? Here are some basic suggestions, which should help you find a new specialist. Also, if you need to change your primary care doctor, these guidelines may assist you, too.

Looking at doctors within your insurance network

Although it's not popular to say anything good about health insurance companies, some of them have thoroughly checked out the doctors that they cover. They often check out malpractice claims, financial records, the doctor's education, and many other aspects of the physicians. They have access to information that's unavailable to most people. They don't want to work with doctors who are lawsuit magnets, and they'll try to screen these doctors out. This is good for patients.

However, some insurance companies merely seek to sign up the doctors who are willing to take a lower payment rate than they would normally accept in order to be in the insurance network. For this reason, sometimes the very best doctors aren't in your particular group or in your health insurance company's "network." As a result, doctors who are "out of network" shouldn't be regarded as inherently risky or bad. Of course, when you're seeking a new primary care doctor or specialist, start within the system of the doctors on your insurance company's list. (Be sure to read more about effective ways of dealing with health insurance companies in Chapter 17.)

If you go "out of network," you may have to pay a higher percentage of the cost, depending on the policy of your health insurance company.

Asking your own doctors who they'd see (or send a family member to)

You've decided that you need to see a specialist for your fibromyalgia, but you have no idea who you'd like to see, so you ask your primary physician to give you a referral. Your primary physician may have dealt personally with a particular specialist before, but don't assume so. Some physicians simply refer their patients to a specialist whom they've heard about through colleagues or they refer you to a specialist who happens to be in the same medical group. You may want to ask your doctor about this specialist and *why* she's referring you to this particular doctor.

In asking your doctors to recommend a specialist, consider asking them the following questions:

✔ What physician would *you* go to see if you had this problem? (Most doctors have been asked this question before, but it may still make them stop and think.)

✔ Would you send your partner, parent, or child to see this doctor? (Similar to the first question, but still a good one to ask because it'll also make most doctors stop and think.)

✔ Have you met this doctor in person or ever talked to him or her at length? (Ideally, your doctor has really met and talked to the doctor that's being recommended. If not, at least you'll know.)

✔ What is it about this doctor that most impresses you? (Listen carefully to the answer and see if it makes sense to you.)

Talking to all your docs

When looking for a new specialist or primary care doctor, ask *all* your doctors (your pediatrician, gynecologist, urologist, or other docs you know) which doctor they would use themselves or send a family member to. Don't restrict yourself to solely asking your internist or family practitioner for a recommendation. Asking different doctors can help to broaden the scope of your search. You may also consider asking other professionals, such as your dentist, whom they would recommend for a chronic pain problem.

Giving docs some basic information about you

Your doctors' recommendations for other doctors will help you narrow down the field. But you should also be sure to provide some basic important information to your doctors beforehand about what you need and want, in order to help them further gauge who to recommend. Ask yourself the following questions and then give the answers to the doctors whose recommendations you seek:

- ✔ How far are you willing to travel to see this doctor? A 20-mile radius? A 50-mile radius? The further you can go, the greater the pool of doctors to choose from.

- ✔ How long are you willing to wait for an appointment? Some doctors may be booked up for months in advance. However, they may be worth the wait.

- ✔ Do you have any special requirements, for example, that you only want to see a female or male doctor or you prefer a doctor of a specific ethnicity? Or do you have some other need? (The pickier you are, the less choices of doctors you'll have.)

- ✔ Must the doctor be on your insurance company's list of approved doctors, or are you willing to pay extra to see an "out of network" physician? It may be worth extra bucks if the new doctor helps you.

Contacting friends and relatives

Many people with fibromyalgia have friends and relatives who also have FMS or are suffering from the apparent symptoms of fibromyalgia. So ask your friends and family members to help you by letting you know if they know of any doctors who've been effective in treating their fibromyalgia or FMS suffered by others they know. You should also keep in mind basic pros and cons of asking family members for help. Also, read Chapter 18 for more information on working with your family when you have FMS.

Here are some pros:

- ✔ They may know many doctors who could help.
- ✔ They may be able to help you get an appointment faster.
- ✔ They may have other ideas on how you can feel better.

And here are some cons:

- ✔ Relatives or friends may try to convince you that you're not really sick.
- ✔ They may be annoyed if you don't see the doctor they like.
- ✔ They may tell everyone else about your problem, and you could get a lot of unwanted advice.

Checking with major medical centers and universities

If you live near a major medical center or in a city with a medical school, in most cases, the doctors there are more likely to be "up" on the latest diagnoses and treatments. They are also more likely to be well informed on fibromyalgia as a pain disorder. This doesn't mean that if you live in the town of Almost Nowhere, your country doctor can't or won't help you. It's just less likely.

Interviewing Your Physician Candidate: What's Up, Doc?

Imagining yourself interviewing a doctor to see whether he or she is right for you can be a pretty scary and daunting thought. Who are you, after all, to be interviewing a smart medical doctor? I'll tell you who you are: a person who needs help and who should find the best doctor you can.

Keep in mind that the United States has thousands of doctors with many different types of medical interests and levels of expertise. What you need is a good "match" between you and your problems and the doctor who will help you to improve your health.

"Doctor shopping" and fibromyalgia

Sometimes, when you see many doctors over a short period of time, you may get the reputation of *doctor shopping*, or looking for a physician who'll give you the answer (or the drug) that you seek. When it comes to people with fibromyalgia, it's hard to *not* appear as if you're doctor shopping when you have to deal with the lack of knowledge that some doctors have about FMS.

As a result, when you see a new doctor for the first time, it's probably a good idea to be very blunt and tell him or her that you're not doctor shopping, but you're looking for someone who can help you feel better. You should avoid proclaiming that nearly every doctor you've ever seen before this time was an idiot or incompetent or a monster. (Even if they were!) Instead, simply say that the previous doctors were unable to help you, for whatever reason. Most doctors can understand and accept that rationale.

When you're thinking about working with a particular doctor, you should definitely consider making an appointment to ask him or her specific questions, even if you have to pay for the appointment. One meeting with the doctor should help you to screen the physician to determine whether he or she may be able to help you.

Here are a few questions to ask prospective physicians. (I also include a few basic guidelines for you to use in evaluating the doctor's answer to each question.)

- ✔ **Is fibromyalgia a prevalent chronic pain syndrome?** If you get a *no* or a convoluted and confusing response, this doctor probably isn't the right one for you. If the doctor says *yes* that fibromyalgia is common, but he adds that he can't be sure that you have FMS, that's an okay and normal answer. The physician is right that he needs to be able to examine you, take a medical history, and rule out other diseases before coming up with a diagnosis. (Read more about this process in Chapter 8.)

- ✔ **Doctor, are you familiar with diagnosing and treating fibromyalgia patients? If so, about how many patients with FMS have you treated?** If it's only one, then don't expect a lot of experience from this doctor. However, many docs are willing to learn about fibromyalgia.

- ✔ **Do your patients with fibromyalgia improve with treatment?** The answer in most cases should be a guarded *yes,* although most physicians know that they don't have any magical cures or talismans to offer people with fibromyalgia. If the doctor's answer is no, that most FMS patients have no hope of improvement, what's the point of spending any time or money with this doctor? You'd better keep looking.

- ✔ **Do you think that you can cure me if I have fibromyalgia?** If you ask the doctor whether he or she thinks that you can be *cured* forever of your fibromyalgia and the answer is an unequivocal **yes,** be very careful about signing up with this doc. Although some physicians may believe that they have the one true answer to the problem, most doctors instead see fibromyalgia as a chronic disease that has its ups and downs.

- ✔ **How long do you think it may take for treatments or medications to make me feel better?** When you ask this question, most doctors will honestly say that they don't know. If the doctor says that you'll be completely cured in just a few weeks or a month, be very dubious about receiving your medical treatment from this person.

    Of course, your doctor may be able to help you quickly alleviate some of your most severe symptoms, particularly the pain and fatigue, with medications or treatments that you may not have tried before. The watchwords are to retain a healthy skepticism and avoid seeking quick fixes.

You're the only one who knows whether this physician has gained your confidence. If you don't feel comfortable with a particular physician, find someone who is more compassionate and skillful. Finding the right doctor for you may take some time, but it's definitely worth the search.

Chapter 8

Getting Physical:
Your Initial Exam and Diagnosis

. . . .

In This Chapter

▶ Understanding what goes into a medical history

▶ Volunteering information when your doctor doesn't ask for it

▶ Identifying the tender points of fibromyalgia

▶ Understanding the necessity of touch in a diagnosis

▶ Testing as part of the diagnostic process

. . . .

*M*any people with fibromyalgia syndrome (FMS) report that they've seen numerous doctors, and obtaining a diagnosis of their illness has taken a year or more. Knowledge is power, and some self-education on the basics of the diagnostic process can help you to help your doctor. Armed with this information, you may be able to shorten the time to reach your diagnosis and treatment.

This chapter tells you about the information-gathering and decision-making process that doctors go through to decide what's wrong with you. You can also find tips on how to talk to your doctor about your symptoms and on how to know when to speak up for yourself. It also covers what tests doctors often use to help them with their diagnosis. In general, laboratory tests and other analyses, such as scans, are negative for people with FMS because doctors use the tests to rule out that another condition or disease is causing the symptom.

Diving into Your Medical History: What the Doctor Should Ask You

Most doctors agree that an integral part of an examination for any new patient is the careful taking of a medical history. *Medical histories* usually involve your past and current medical problems as well as any surgeries that you may have had and medications that you currently take. If you're a new patient, you'll nearly always be given a form to fill out regarding this information, or the doctor or a nurse will ask you the questions directly. In fact, even if you've seen the doctor before, it's still a good idea for the physician to perform (or have the nurse perform) at least a quick review of your medical history. Doctors can use this information to check for patterns or clues to help them with your current diagnosis.

You can't possibly know exactly what your physician needs to know to diagnose you. So, rather than trying to screen your answers, just answer all the questions honestly, even if they don't seem important to you, and leave it up to the physician to figure out how to use the information. Provide complete and accurate answers. Something that may seem unimportant to you, such as an operation you had ten years ago, could be relevant to the doctor.

If you have fibromyalgia or think that you may have it, and you've told the doctor about your diagnosis (or your suspicion that you may have fibromyalgia), the doctor should also ask you questions that relate to FMS. Here are a few examples of FMS-type questions that may be asked, although don't expect the doctor to follow my exact wording like a script!

Setting diagnostic criteria for FMS

In 1990, the American College of Rheumatology, a professional organization of thousands of rheumatologists, developed criteria to help doctors determine whether their patients had fibromyalgia. Many (but not all) doctors of all specialties, as well as general practitioners, use these guidelines to help them with their diagnoses. Very basically, these following criteria were offered to doctors:

✔ Widespread musculoskeletal pain for at least three months on both the right and left sides of the body

✔ Pain both above and below the waist (for example, in the neck and buttock area)

✔ Pain experienced when at least 11 of 18 specified tender points (check out Figure 8-1, which illustrates these tender points) are touched with a force of about 9 pounds or less

✔ Other symptoms, such as sleep disorders and muscle stiffness

- ✔ Does the pain change in intensity, sometimes getting a lot worse or a lot better?

- ✔ Does the pain move around, or is it primarily in the same place all the time?

- ✔ Do you have morning stiffness? Do you also have stiffness throughout the day? (Most FMS patients have some level of muscle pain.)

- ✔ Do you have trouble sleeping? If so, about how many hours a night do you think that you're sleeping? (Sleep problems are very common among people who have fibromyalgia.)

- ✔ Are you experiencing extreme fatigue, beyond the normal tiredness many people have?

Volunteering Info if the Doc Doesn't Ask You

In most cases, the doctor will ask you questions that elicit the information that's needed to give you good treatment. Once in awhile, however, some facts or complaints may not come out in the course of your encounter with your doctor. Be sure to volunteer any information that you think may be important.

Whatever happens, make sure that you accomplish the principal mission of your office visit: Communicate your chief medical complaints to your doctor. You may find that, for example, the doctor seems primarily concerned about your insufficient sleep and is concentrating on that problem. But you may feel instead that you're being driven mad by the pain you're suffering from. *Tell* the doctor about your distress with the pain and that it bothers you the most.

Don't wait until the end of your doctor's visit to tell your physician what's really bothering you. "Oh, doctor, I just remembered, I have excruciating pain that goes from my neck to my back, and I also have been passing out a lot." I'm exaggerating for emphasis (fainting isn't a usual symptom of fibromyalgia), but, sometimes, patients really do hold off on revealing extremely important information until the doctor is ready to walk out. Don't make this mistake because if you do, you'll be shortchanging yourself by not accentuating your most troubling symptoms or problems early on when the doctor has time to consider possible causes as well as solutions that may help you.

In fact, it's a very good idea to write down two or three key points on a piece of paper ahead of time and to bring it with you to your appointment. Why? Because you may very easily forget what you'd meant to ask the doctor, and you may find that you remember your questions only after you've driven all the way home again. Of course, you shouldn't bring a scroll of complaints with you to the doctor's office. Keep your list short and simple.

Pay particular attention to volunteering information about your pain, other doctors you're currently seeing, and medications, vitamins, and supplements that you're taking.

Grinning and bearing it: An unadvisable way to go

Don't assume that your doctor will somehow automatically know that your pain is very severe. Although most physicians are very smart and very dedicated people who really want to help their patients feel better, they don't have an internal "psychic hotline" that enables them to read minds and magically know how people feel or what's distressing them the most. So please don't assume that your doctor will always know (or should know) what's bothering you or what you really need or want. Tell her. Also, try to provide details. Pain can be hard to describe. But is it a burning kind of pain? A pressure pain? A stabbing pain? Provide as many details as possible, so that your doctor can help you resolve your pain problem.

If your pain has become extreme, you may be experiencing another medical problem. Even if it *is* your FMS that's causing you to hurt so badly, severe pain requires treatment. So speak up.

Laying out common mistakes patients make during physical exams

You want to get better, don't you? Of course, you do! But you may inadvertently make one or more of the common errors that can impair your diagnosis. Do you:

✔ Tell the doctor that you know what's wrong with you because your mother's friend's cousin said that she has the exact same thing, and her doctor said it was _____ (fill in the blank)?

Doctors can get really aggravated when people assume that a non-physician can make an accurate diagnosis. If a birth relative, such as a parent or sibling, has similar problems, tell the doctor. But let the physician make the diagnostic call.

✔ Spend a lot of time on "small talk"?

Pleasantries are nice but the doctor's time is usually very limited. Get to the point as soon as possible. Why are you here, and what do you hope the doctor will do for you?

✔ Withhold information?

If you're doing something that you think the doctor will disapprove of (such as drinking, smoking, taking drugs, or some other behavior), tell him anyway. These behaviors can have a direct impact on your diagnosis as well as your treatment. Sure, the doctor may tell you to stop these behaviors. But, well, shouldn't you stop them?

Seeing other doctors

If you're seeing other doctors in addition to the one who's diagnosing you, tell the doctor about it. Physicians need to know about other doctors you see in case they have any questions that need to be followed up with those other doctors.

Doctors prescribe medication — that's a fact of life. The diagnosing doc also needs to know about all the other doctors in your life because she needs to know about all the medicines that you're taking — not just the ones she's prescribed for you.

Bringing your medications with you

If any other doctor has prescribed medications or recommended over-the-counter medications for you, bring them along with you to your doctor's appointment in the original prescription bottle or over-the-counter container. Why? Because forgetting the dosage of your medicines is very easy — many people do. And doctors really hate it when patients say, "It's the little blue pill, I forgot the name." Do you know how many little blue pills are out there? Too many!

The doctor won't want to prescribe a medicine for you that may interact badly when taken in combination with a drug that you already take. To avoid that problem, the physician must first know what other medicines you're taking now. You know what you're taking, so share that information.

Drugs that you buy in the health food store or over the counter at the pharmacy are still drugs, even if you don't need a prescription to buy them. As a result, "natural" and over-the-counter drugs can interfere with or prevent other drugs that you're taking from working properly. So do be sure to tell your doctor. Or better yet — show him.

Adding on vitamins or supplements

Many people with fibromyalgia are in such pain that they're willing to try virtually anything to feel better — including questionable treatments, some of which may include taking vitamins and supplements (Read Chapter 12, which deals with alternative remedies, for some of the useful treatments as well as some of the strange ones that people have selected.)

Patients have nearly died (and some patients *have* died) because they failed to tell their doctor about a "natural" drug they were taking. You really need to inform your doctor about everything that you're taking because whatever medicines you're taking now may affect your laboratory results. It could also cause a serious interaction with a medication that the doctor might prescribe, unaware of what you're already on.

Some types of supplements may bring you some relief. For example, if a person is deficient in a mineral like magnesium or calcium, in that case, a supplement makes sense. But you really can't *know* if you're deficient in any vitamins or minerals unless your doctor tests you, so you should avoid taking vitamins and supplements unless your doctor says that you need them. Many supplements present risks of varying degrees. For example, if you take too much Vitamin C, you can cause gastrointestinal upset. If you take too much magnesium, you may inadvertently create a potassium deficiency or other deficiency. So, instead of simply telling your doctor what vitamins and supplements you're taking, the best course of action is to consult with her before you start taking any of these substances.

Getting All Your Questions Out in the Open

Some people believe that if any information is important, the doctor will automatically provide it to them. Based on that belief, they don't ask questions and are passive patients. But doctors *can't* always know exactly what you're most concerned about or what you don't understand. That's why asking questions is important. Don't be shy! If you don't understand something or your doctor hasn't covered the topic that you're most keen on knowing about, just ask her.

If you're concerned that maybe the doctor wasn't listening to you or didn't hear something you said that was important, don't agonize within your mind about whether she did or didn't hear you. Just say it again. Make sure that the doctor is looking at you when you say it and isn't jotting down notes, talking on the phone, or doing some other multitasking thing. To get the doc's attention, say her name and wait until she looks at you. If necessary, say the name *again*, even if it's when she's walking out the door. "Dr. Smith, I have one more question!" If the doctor has a name that's hard to pronounce, use the first letter of the last name. "Dr. Z., I need to know . . ." Most people, including doctors, find it hard to ignore people who are calling them by name.

Identifying the Tender Points of Fibromyalgia

Another very important part of the diagnosis of fibromyalgia, after ruling out other medical problems that you may have had, is for physicians to consider whether or not you have tender points. In fact, the existence of tender points is one of the hallmarks that helps doctors to diagnose fibromyalgia.

Tender points, a key diagnostic feature of fibromyalgia, are specific areas of the body that are very painful when gently probed. (Tender points aren't the same as *trigger points,* also covered in Chapter 6, which are lumpy or ropey muscular knots or inflammations.) With tender points, the patient feels the pain, but the doctor can't feel any apparent abnormalities or detect the presence of inflammation or disease. When the problem is fibromyalgia, the doctor typically sees nothing unusual about the body except for the reaction of the patient, who typically winces or cringes.

Some patients find out about their tender points for the first time during an office visit. For example, Lucy learned about tender points in a very un-tender way. But first, here's some background on Lucy. She says that for years, every time she saw any doctor, she asked the physician to explain to her why she was so sore in the area that would be covered by an elbow-length shirt — most of her upper body (neck, arms, back, chest). But none of the doctors seemed to know or care.

Then one day, Lucy was seeing her family doctor, and she asked him if he thought that she might have fibromyalgia. He suddenly and very unexpectedly poked her hard in one of the tender spots between her neck and shoulder. It was so painful that Lucy screamed, and she says that she nearly passed out. How did the doctor react? He told her *yes,* she did have fibromyalgia. Fortunately, most doctors aren't as insensitive as Lucy's (former!) doctor was.

Touching is part of the process

Doctors need to touch their patients in most physical examinations, if only to check their basic reflexes. But touching the patient is even more important if a person may have fibromyalgia because physical pain is a key problem faced by most people with FMS. The doctor needs to see if it hurts when you're touched, where it hurts, and how much it hurts.

If you try to be really brave and avoid wincing or reacting at all when the doctor presses a tender point, or any other part of your body that hurts, how can he or she know that it hurts? You shouldn't try to play Ms. or Mr. Stoic. Wincing is okay. In fact, you may find it hard not to.

Locating your tender points

The 18 tender points that doctors use to help them diagnose fibromyalgia (as developed by the American College of Rheumatology) are primarily located on the upper torso, although a few can be found on other parts of the body, such as in the knees. Check out Figure 8-1 for a drawing of the location of these tender points. All these tender points add up to a grand total of 18. And according to the guidelines established by the American College of Rheumatology, to obtain an official diagnosis of fibromyalgia, you must feel pain in 11 or more of them. (For more info regarding these guidelines, check out the "Setting diagnostic criteria for FMS" sidebar in this chapter.) Hopefully, you won't feel pain in all 18 places!

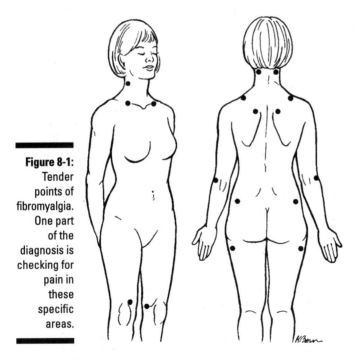

Figure 8-1:
Tender
points of
fibromyalgia.
One part
of the
diagnosis is
checking for
pain in
these
specific
areas.

Of course, people with fibromyalgia frequently have pain that's not limited to these 18 areas. Consequently, if you hurt elsewhere, that pain's probably from your fibromyalgia, too. The specific tender points were selected by doctors as most characteristic of people with FMS, which is why they're often used in the diagnostic process.

Assigning a tender number to FMS

According to the American College of Rheumatology, a person should have some pain in at least 11 of the 18 tender points to be diagnosed with fibromyalgia. Some doctors follow this guideline while others think that if you have 9 or 10 tender points (or even fewer) but you meet other criteria, you may have fibromyalgia.

The presence of many tender points indicates a high probability that fibromyalgia exists — if other medical problems have been ruled out and if the person also exhibits other symptoms of FMS, such as severe fatigue or difficulty with insomnia or other sleep problems. Whether or not the doctor is a stickler for a given number of tender points as a cutoff really depends on the physician.

Rheumatologists are probably the most likely to consider tender points as very important because rheumatologists were the ones who devised this criteria and also because it's quantitative data in an area where hard data and verification aren't easy to come by.

One problem with using tender points as mandatory diagnostic criteria is that fibromyalgia is a very changeable syndrome. As a result, most people who have fibromyalgia feel better on some days and worse on others. This inconsistency means that some people who really do have fibromyalgia may only "score" with 9 or 10 tender points on a given day, but the following week, they could have pain in all 18 tender point areas.

It also means that if patients see their doctors on the day they have less than 11 tender points and the physicians are very rigid about the tender points criteria, some cases of FMS won't be diagnosed.

Test-ifying About FMS

Most of the tests that doctors order when they think that you may have fibromyalgia are really tests for other medical problems. Although doctors should take a hard look at the symptoms you exhibit, they can't say for sure that you have fibromyalgia until they're able to rule those other diseases and conditions out. FMS has no specific tests, other than the tender points criteria described earlier. In the future, doctors may test you for hormones and other body chemicals that may be higher or lower when you have fibromyalgia. But that's not happening right now.

Ordering up a round of lab tests

Part of your physical examination may include laboratory tests, such as blood tests and urinalysis. It's normal for the doctor to want such tests to be done, and you shouldn't be alarmed if your doctor orders them.

Ruling out autoimmune disorders

The pain of fibromyalgia may appear to the doctor to be the beginnings of *rheumatoid arthritis* or *lupus*, both very serious and deteriorating arthritic conditions. Another possibility is *multiple sclerosis*, also a serious disease. In addition, the doctor will often want to verify that you don't have a thyroid disease. *Hypothyroidism*, or below normal levels of thyroid hormone, can also cause fatigue and muscle and joint pain. Sometimes these conditions can coexist with fibromyalgia.

These diseases are known as *autoimmune disorders,* or diseases resulting from the body's immune system actually attacking itself. A blood test will reveal if your blood includes a special "factor" that indicates that you may have rheumatoid arthritis or lupus. If the blood test comes back "negative," you're unlikely to have them. A spinal fluid examination can detect antibodies that are characteristic of multiple sclerosis.

How do doctors diagnose people?

In general, most doctors diagnose patients with a process that is called a *differential diagnosis*, which means that they consider all the possible things that might be wrong with you, based on your symptoms, gender, age, geographic location, and other factors. They then narrow the diagnosis down to the most likely one.

For example, if you're a woman living in Peoria, Illinois, you're unlikely to have malaria. If you are a man, you flat out *will not* have menstrual problems. For possible fibromyalgia sufferers, the doctor considers the location of your pain/discomfort to aid with the diagnosis. If you're suffering from painful cramps in your toes, you may have fibromyalgia. But you may also have a vitamin deficiency or a problem with dehydration. Laboratory tests help the doctor rule out other medical problems and further narrow down the list to what is most likely.

A blood test can also measure the level of circulating thyroid hormone. If your levels are out of range, you're *hypothyroid* (low thyroid levels) or *hyperthyroid* (excessively high levels of thyroid hormone). The doctor can also check a sedimentation rate to identify inflammation, and he can order a chemistry panel, which will show how well (or poorly) your kidneys and liver are functioning.

Excluding blood diseases

The doctor will also often order a *complete blood count* (CBC), which is a count of your red and white blood cells. It's also a check on whether you might have a blood disease that can cause a person to feel weak and achy, such as anemia or another blood disease. If the CBC comes back normal, in most cases, you don't have such a disease. The doctor will also usually order a test of your blood glucose to rule out *diabetes* (characterized by *hyperglycemia*, or high levels of blood glucose) or, at the other end of the scale, *hypoglycemia*, a condition of unusually low blood sugar.

Verifying it's not a vitamin deficiency

Blood tests can also verify if you're deficient in any major vitamins or minerals, such as Vitamin B_{12} or calcium, magnesium, potassium, or other minerals. A vitamin or mineral shortage can cause pain and weakness.

Sometimes, people who take medications for an illness can develop a vitamin or mineral deficiency, which leads to side effects and symptoms. For example, people with high blood pressure (also known as *hypertension*) may need medication, which can lead to a side effect of depleting the body of potassium.

The person suffering from a potassium deficiency may be able to just eat a few bananas a day to make up for this deficiency, or he or she may need to take supplemental potassium every day to reach normalcy. The blood tests that you have will show whether you have a deficiency and, if one is present, how severe it is.

Counting out infectious illnesses

The same CBC that the doc uses to rule out blood diseases can also show whether you may have an infection because your white blood cell count will be slightly (or very much) higher than normal — although usually not dangerously higher than normal, as found with a blood disease.

The doctor should also screen your blood for hepatitis C, which may cause fibromyalgia-like symptoms. (Read more about this problem in Chapter 3.)

Doctors may also test for Lyme disease, particularly for patients who live in the northeastern parts of the United States. (Read more about Lyme disease, which is a diagnosis sometimes confused with FMS, in Chapter 6.)

In addition, the urine can be checked for possible kidney disease. High levels of protein in the urine (also known as *proteinuria*) or of other elements that are not normally present may indicate the beginning of a kidney disease that needs to be treated.

Considering CT scans or MRIs

In some cases, the doctor will decide that you need a special scan of the part of your body that's causing you pain. The physician may order a high-tech x-ray, known as the *computerized tomography* (CT) scan, or she may order a *magnetic resonance imaging* (MRI) test. The doctor may also order regular x-rays, if he or she thinks that you may have arthritis or other bone changes.

Neither the CT scan nor the MRI (nor plain x-rays) is invasive nor do these tests cause any pain. However, some people are disturbed by the noise generated by the MRI. Because people with fibromyalgia can be hypersensitive to noise, they're also more likely to be distressed by the MRI. Many MRI technicians offer a solution to this problem by giving you headphones to listen to music during the procedure.

For some people, another potential issue with having an MRI is that your body is enclosed in a small area. If you suffer from *claustrophobia*, or anxiety or fear about being in confined spaces, you may want to ask the doctor to give you a mild sedative before you have the MRI. Of course, if you do take a sedative, you'll need someone to drive you there and then drive you home afterwards. In some cases, your doctor may be able to order an open-sided MRI for you, avoiding the problem of claustrophobia, although not all insurance companies cover the use of this equipment.

Doctors use MRIs, CT scans, and x-rays to rule out a number of possibilities:

- **Bone diseases:** The x-rays, CT scan, or MRI will check for any fractures or abnormalities of the skeletal system, such as caused by arthritis or other diseases. And yes, you can have a minor fracture and still be walking around — although you probably won't be walking perfectly normally and you'll have at least some pain.

- **Other diseases:** An MRI can also rule out some diseases, such as multiple sclerosis.

- **Brain abnormalities:** These tests can rule out problems, such as a brain tumor or aneurysm (tiny blood vessel about to burst).

- **Organic problems:** One or more of your major organs may be malfunctioning, anywhere from your thyroid gland to your colon to any other organ in any system of your body.

Using ultrasound for diagnosis

An *ultrasound* is a special device that uses sound waves to create outlines of an organ, and along with other tests, it can be helpful with diagnosis. Pregnant women usually have at least one or two ultrasounds of their baby during the course of the pregnancy, so that the obstetrician can make sure that the fetus is developing normally. The ultrasound isn't invasive and is usually not painful, unless the ultrasound wand is pressed against an area of the body that's hurting. The ultrasound technician will be as gentle as possible.

An ultrasound can detect the following:

✔ **Organic abnormalities:** The doctor will usually order the ultrasound to check areas of the body that are most prone to problems. For example, could you have a problem with your gall bladder, stomach, or colon? A combination of the physical examination, your answers to the doctor's questions, and the laboratory tests and ultrasound will together help rule out organic abnormalities that are causing your medical problem.

✔ **Tissue/nerve problems:** Is there inflammation? With fibromyalgia, patients do *not* have any inflammation that's detectable in standard laboratory tests. If your ultrasound reveals inflammation or tissue damage, you have another medical problem rather than (or in addition to) fibromyalgia. Many doctors will perform a neurological exam, which includes testing of your reflexes and your responses to pressure and touch. It may also be important to test your muscle strength because some rare muscle diseases can mimic fibromyalgia.

Part III

Getting to Wellness: How Fibromyalgia is Treated

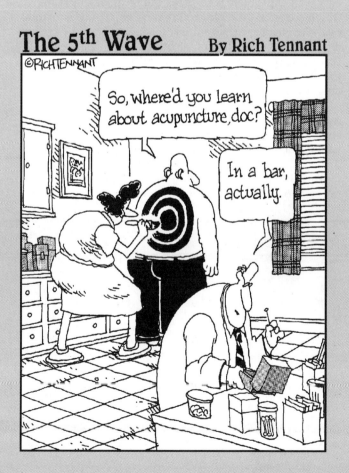

The 5th Wave   By Rich Tennant

So, where'd you learn about acupuncture, doc?

In a bar, actually.

In this part . . .

After you know that you really *have* fibromyalgia,
you'll want to know what on earth to do about this
aggravating problem, and that's the purpose of Part III,
which covers a wide range of treatment options. I include
over-the-counter drugs, under-the-counter drugs (just kidding; I mean prescribed medications), and what I call
"hands-on therapy," which is basically therapy that
touches your skin and muscles such as icing and heating,
massage therapy, mud baths, and other options.

And I don't forget alternative remedies! Some good (and
some less-than-good) alternative remedies exist for people
with fibromyalgia, and I cover the gamut. I review supplements, acupuncture, botox injections, aromatherapy,
magnet therapy, and a few other intriguing choices. I offer
my candid, expert opinion on each option.

Chapter 9

Medicating the Problem: Over-the-Counter Drugs May Help

In This Chapter

▶ Regarding guaifenesin

▶ Optimizing over-the-counter painkillers

▶ Considering antihistamines or cold remedies that may help

▶ Talking about topical remedies

T ina says that she feels so much better since she's started taking guaifenesin to treat her fibromyalgia. According to Tina, she still has plenty of back pain, fatigue, and other symptoms of fibromyalgia syndrome (FMS). But compared to how she felt *before* she began the "guaifenesin protocol," Tina says that she's radically better. Marcy, on the other hand, has been taking guaifenesin faithfully for two years, and she says she's yet to see any results whatsoever. But Marcy figures that the positive effects should kick in anytime now, as long as she's very patient, so she's continuing to take the drug. Tom took guaifenesin for about a month, but didn't notice any improvement in his condition, so he gave up on it.

Guaifenesin (guai rhymes with "may" and *fenesin* rhymes with "venison" or "Tennyson") is a cough medicine that's currently being promoted by some patients and doctors as a treatment for fibromyalgia, but taking a popularity poll on over-the-counter drugs to decide what you take isn't a good idea at all. Anecdotal recommendations are usually worthy of consideration, when it comes to finding a plumber or even a physician. But I think that a far better way to consider whether to take medications, such as guaifenesin, as well as other over-the-counter (nonprescribed) remedies to treat fibromyalgia, is to look at existing clinical studies, as well as to consider patient comments. I provide both objective data and subjective anecdotal information on guaifenesin in this chapter.

I include guaifenesin as an *over-the-counter* (OTC) drug, because it's available in an OTC strength, and many people who take it rely on OTC guaifenesin. An over-the-counter drug is a medication that doesn't require a prescription from your doctor, but it's still regulated by the Food and Drug Administration (FDA). OTC medications must receive approval from the FDA before they can be introduced, and the FDA can pull them off the market if problems develop. However, guaifenesin is also available in a prescribed strength, as are some of the other medications described in this chapter.

In this chapter, I also cover antihistamines (cold medicine-type remedies), painkilling remedies (such as Tylenol, aspirin, and ibuprofen), and topical pain-relief remedies (ointments, creams, and so on that you can rub into your skin, hopefully allowing you at least a temporary reprieve from your pain).

Examining the Nuts and Bolts of Guaifenesin

Guaifenesin is an *expectorant,* which is a drug that thins out and loosens your mucous, making the mucous easier to cough up. Guaifenesin is also one of the ingredients that's often found in popular cough syrups; however, individuals who support taking guaifenesin for the symptoms of fibromyalgia believe that it's best to take guaifenesin alone, without these other added drugs.

Some guaifenesin supporters take an over-the-counter dose of the drug; others take a prescribed level. Some individuals supplement their prescription guaifenesin with OTC guaifenesin. And still others manage to take a prescription-level dose of guaifenesin by taking a lot of OTC guaifenesin tablets. I don't recommend this practice at all because I believe that your doctor should monitor prescribed drug strengths. It can be very dangerous to take high doses of OTC drugs, and people have accidentally died this way. It is wrong and can be harmful to act on the mistaken belief that if two pills would be good (as recommended on the bottle), then four would be twice as good.

Guaifenesin is not an FDA-approved treatment for fibromyalgia. So far, clinical studies have *not* proven that guaifenesin is an effective treatment for people who have fibromyalgia or any other ailment beyond a serious cough or chronic asthma. (Take a look at the "Studying guaifenesin" section in this chapter for some info on the one clinical study of guaifenesin.) So what's the real deal on "guai," as its proponents affectionately like to call it?

Looking at some background info

Guaifenesin as a solution to fibromyalgia was the brainchild of Dr. Paul St. Amand, an endocrinologist from California. Guaifenesin has been used for many years to treat people's coughs. So why do some proponents fervently believe that this drug can now help them alleviate their symptoms of fibromyalgia?

Dr. R. Paul St. Amand, the number-one advocate of using guaifenesin to treat fibromyalgia, believes that people with fibromyalgia build up caches of chemicals (phosphates) in their bodies. He believes that these deposits result in the pain and other symptoms that are characteristic of fibromyalgia.

Dr. St. Amand also strongly believes, based on personal and anecdotal observations of his own patients, that the regular taking of guaifenesin can slowly rid the body of these chemical deposits, and, consequently, will eventually make patients with fibromyalgia feel dramatically better. Or so the theory goes. Some people are said to feel well more quickly than others, and supposedly, some patients may have to wait a year or longer before they gain noticeable benefits from taking the drug.

Studying guaifenesin

Physicians who are aware of the use of guaifenesin to treat fibromyalgia apparently have mixed feelings about this remedy. Some doctors take a neutral stance about the use of guaifenesin, and others are more negative, saying that because the use of guaifenesin isn't backed up by clinical studies, it should never be used to treat fibromyalgia. Other physicians believe that if the drug doesn't cause identifiable harm, it's okay for patients with FMS to try it, as long as competent doctors are carefully following the patients.

Clinical studies to date haven't backed up the use of guaifenesin as a treatment for fibromyalgia. Dr. Robert Bennett, a highly respected rheumatologist and clinical researcher in Oregon, performed a one-year clinical study on guaifenesin among 40 women who were diagnosed with fibromyalgia. (The study wasn't published in a journal, but as of this writing, it's available at www.myalgia.com/guaif2.htm.)

Dr. Bennett subsequently concluded that guaifenesin didn't significantly improve the subjects' symptoms of fibromyalgia, compared to the effects of the placebo (sugar pill) on the control group.

Dr. St. Armand, who was an advisor to the researchers of the clinical study, has since ardently disputed the study findings. But to date, no other clinical studies have been performed that support or refute Dr. Bennett's research. No on can definitively state that guaifenesin doesn't help fibromyalgia, based on just one study that refutes its value. Nor can anyone say with certainty that guaifenesin helps the symptoms of FMS, based on the views of Dr. St. Armand and some anecdotal reports of success. The only thing that's absolutely clear is that further studies are needed. But guaifenesin's adoring fans abound.

Joining the fan club

Although guaifenesin has no clinical proof that it works, it does have a lot of anecdotal evidence that the drug helps some patients. These testimonials come from many individuals who are convinced that guaifenesin has played a major role in their improvement.

For example, Susan, a long-time sufferer of fibromyalgia syndrome (FMS), says that guaifenesin has given her back a semblance of a normal life — one she thought had been lost to her forever. Last year, Susan says that she could barely climb a flight of stairs, and she had to take them one at a time, like a toddler who's just learned how to walk. But now, she goes up and down the stairs several times a day effortlessly, the way most adults unthinkingly use stairs.

Diana, another person who's had fibromyalgia for years, agrees completely with Susan about the effectiveness of guaifenesin and is another ardent proponent. Diana says that since she started taking guaifenesin, her pain has been reduced by about 80 percent, and her fatigue is about half of what she suffered from before. Because pain and fatigue were her two prevailing symptoms, she's become a true believer in the value of taking daily doses of guaifenesin.

Kathy is another fibromyalgia sufferer, and she says that she's taken at least 30 different medications for her fibromyalgia. Kathy says that none of these drugs helped her, and that the only drug that has given her any symptomatic relief whatsoever has been guaifenesin.

Susan, Diana, and Kathy are only three of many people who believe that guaifenesin has been a life changer for them. However, others say that guaifenesin hasn't helped them at all, or that the drug has made them feel worse.

 If you want to contact very strong and committed supporters of the use of guaifenesin and you'd like to find out their detailed information about its use in treating fibromyalgia, you can go to a Web site of a support group at `www.netromall.com/guai-support`. Or you may want to go directly to the source of the doctor who promotes guaifenesin as a therapy for fibromyalgia at `www.guaidoc.com`.

Ordering guaifenesin

If you decide that you want to try guaifenesin, despite the lack of clinical studies to support its use in fibromyalgia, you may have a hard time finding the drug by itself in your local drugstore because it's usually one ingredient among others in OTC cold remedies. However, you can ask your pharmacist to order you an OTC dose of guaifenesin alone.

You can also order an OTC dose of guaifenesin over the Internet, but generally, you're better off working with your local pharmacist. Some sites even offer prescribed doses of guaifenesin, but you should definitely stay away from them. State Medical Boards strongly disapprove of doctors and pharmacies who prescribe drugs for people they have no direct personal relationship with, because they're worried about possible overdoses or side effects.

Pondering the guaifenesin protocol

If you decide that guaifenesin may be the answer to diminishing the effects of your fibromyalgia symptoms, you may want to follow the "guaifenesin protocol." This plan is very complicated, and it requires careful thought. A key aspect of this protocol involves taking guaifenesin indefinitely. Its proponents compare the continued taking of guaifenesin to the need people with other chronic illnesses have to take medication for life.

For example, people with hypertension must continue to take blood pressure pills even when their blood pressure is down, just as individuals with other chronic diseases must also continue to take other medications.

Mapping your body's bumps

One key feature of guaifenesin protocol is "mapping" the lumps and bumps of your entire body before you start taking the drug for comparison purposes after you've been taking guaifenesin for awhile. These lumps and bumps are considered to be contracted (spastic) muscles and are completely different from the *tender points* of fibromyalgia defined by the American College of Rheumatology, as discussed in Chapter 8. Tender points hurt the patient when pressed, but the doctor can't feel anything. In contrast, the bumps described by supporters of using guaifenesin are not considered symptoms of fibromyalgia by most physicians.

Mapping is supposedly best performed by a physician, although finding a doctor who's willing or able to do this task may be very difficult. Most doctors know nothing about mapping, nor will they take the time to learn it or perform it on all their patients who have fibromyalgia. As a result, some patients ask their chiropractor, massage therapist, or other individuals who are experienced in treating muscle pain to learn the process of mapping and perform that task on them. Some people watch a videotape on mapping and manage to perform their own personal evaluation of their bodies.

After the mapping is performed, the guaifenesin regimen is launched. At some point in the future, the body is mapped again, to determine whether some of those lumps or bumps have disappeared. If so, this evidence supposedly proves that the guaifenesin worked.

The problem with this concept, however, is that people's bodies change over time, and some benign lumps or bumps that are here today may naturally disappear by themselves at a later date. Also, if a medical doctor doesn't perform the precise mapping, the practice itself seems suspect.

Please don't take guaifenesin on your own without discussing it with your doctor. Combined with other medications that you may take, or with other medical problems that you may have, guaifenesin may be an inadvisable drug for you.

Avoiding aspirin

Avoiding drugs or cosmetics that include salicylates (aspirin-containing substances) and meeting other very detailed criteria are also important parts of the guaifenesin protocol to those who support it. It's all spelled out for you in excruciating detail in a book written by Dr. St. Armand. If you choose to follow this regimen, be prepared to spend a great deal of time figuring it all out. Of course, if it works, it will be worth a major investment of time and planning.

Riding a cycle

Another key part of the theory behind recommending guaifenesin to people with fibromyalgia is that people will periodically feel much worse, which guaifenesin proponents refer to as cycling. *Cycling* is supposedly proof that you're ridding your body of phosphates, those chemicals that had theoretically clogged your body so much that your kidneys couldn't excrete them all.

Cycling is said to be a painful process, in the sense that your fibromyalgia symptoms worsen. People who are supposedly in the midst of "cycling" are often urged by guaifenesin proponents to tough it out because they believe that a time when you'll feel much better is in the near future.

The problem with the cycling concept is that no clinical proof states that it actually happens. The one study performed on guaifenesin as a therapy for fibromyalgia tested the urine of patients to see if they were excreting substances that could be considered as phosphates. They weren't. So far, there's no quantitative way to determine if and when cycling is occurring.

Many people taking guaifenesin think that they're cycling because they feel worse. But here's the thing: People with fibromyalgia who *don't* take guaifenesin also experience some periods when they feel much worse, too, with their symptoms becoming much more troublesome. If the nonguaifenesin patients aren't cycling, what's happening? It's probably the normal ups and downs of a chronic disease.

Weighing the pros and cons of guaifenesin

I offer a brief overview of the advantages and disadvantages of guaifenesin use as a treatment for fibromyalgia.

Accentuating the positives

Simply put, here are the basic advantages of guaifenesin treatment (other than that its supporters fervently believe that it makes them feel much better):

- ✔ It's generally an inexpensive medication.
- ✔ It's often relatively easy to obtain.
- ✔ Guaifenesin has few or no side effects for most users, although some side effects are listed later in this chapter and also in Appendix B.
- ✔ You won't need a prescription for the low doses of the drug.

  However, if you decide that you want to take higher doses of guaifenesin than are readily available in the over-the-counter medications (as recommended by many people who advocate taking guaifenesin for fibromyalgia symptoms), you'll have to take a few extra OTC pills (which I don't recommend at all), or you'll need to ask your doctor to give you a prescription for the higher dosage medication.

Looking at the drawbacks

The key disadvantage of taking guaifenesin is that it may not make you feel any better at all. Generally, people like the medications they take to actually work for them, although the harsh reality is that, many times, medications don't help particular individuals. But the only way to know whether some drugs work is to take them and see what happens. You may keep on taking the drug, and *still* not feel any better.

Another disadvantage is that many people who strongly support the taking of guaifenesin won't believe you if you say that it's not helping you. They *know* in their hearts that it's the right drug because they strongly support guaifenesin as a kind of fibromyalgia salvation. These individuals may tell you that if guaifenesin isn't working for you, it's somehow your own fault — you're not taking enough of the drug or maybe you're doing something else that's plain wrong. Many proponents apparently assume that if you were doing it "right," guaifenesin would invariably make you feel much better. They see guaifenesin as a one-drug-fits-all kind of remedy. If you rely on such views, you could find yourself in a confused or self-blaming state — neither of which is helpful.

Along the same lines, hard-core guai supporters will tell you the drug is working regardless of how and what you feel. Ironically, if you find that you feel *worse* when you take guaifenesin, guai supporters believe that feeling worse is "proof" that the drug's working for you because it's allegedly actively ridding your body of pain-inducing chemicals, such as phosphates. (I discuss this "cycling" process in more detail in the section, "Riding a cycle," earlier in this chapter.) If you feel better, that's also a sign that the drug's working. And if you don't feel anything, don't worry. Supposedly, you'll soon feel better or worse, and then you'll know that it's working.

Although guaifenesin has few side effects, some people do have bad reactions to it. Here are some of the more common reactions:

 ✔ The drug may cause skin itching and rashes.

 ✔ It sometimes causes nausea and vomiting.

 ✔ Guaifenesin may also cause drowsiness in some individuals.

 ✔ Some people say that it exacerbates their symptoms of fibromyalgia.

Pulling it all together

The proponents of using guaifenesin to treat fibromyalgia believe that it's working whether you feel nothing, feel worse, or feel better. This is a sort of "Heads I win, tails you lose" kind of thinking, and it can be really quite maddening to physicians like me who have to stick to rigorous rules of clinical research when we perform studies.

Also, I wonder how many patients would be willing to adhere to the same type of regimen if their medical doctor prescribed it. How many people would take a medicine their doctor recommended, for months or even years, when they experienced little or no improvement? Many doctors have a hard enough time getting patients to take their antibiotics for seven days.

I suspect that some of the glamour of guaifenesin is that it's not a mainstream remedy. If many doctors suddenly urged their patients to take guaifenesin for fibromyalgia, I suspect that it might quickly lose much of its allure.

I think that so far, until further studies are performed that support its use, guaifenesin is an unproven remedy for fibromyalgia. I've no evidence that the drug will help *any* of your fibromyalgia symptoms, despite the strong belief by some proponents that it's a form of fibromyalgia salvation.

On the other hand, I don't see guaifenesin as a dangerous drug. If you consult with your physician on the use of the drug and your doctor agrees that you can try and see if it eases any of your FMS symptoms, generally, trying guaifenesin won't hurt you. Guaifenesin may have some mild analgesic qualities, as well as some mild muscle-relaxing capabilities.

I still can't rule out guaifenesin as a possible remedy for fibromyalgia until further studies are performed, but I can't support it as a sure-fire remedy, either.

Relieving Pain with Painkillers

Your doctor may prescribe painkilling medications or other types of drugs to help you cope with the aching, stiffness, and the overall pain of fibromyalgia.

(Read Chapter 10 for more information on prescribed medications.) But if your symptoms have lessened somewhat and yet at the same time, you still feel bad enough that you need to take something for pain relief, an over-the-counter painkilling medication may be the right answer for you. Here are a few options:

- **Acetaminophen:** You probably know this drug by a different name, Tylenol.

  The simple short-term benefit of taking over-the-counter Tylenol is that it may give you some a temporary respite from your widespread body aches and pains. Many people see Tylenol as extremely safe, and it generally *is* a safe medication. However, long-term and heavy use of Tylenol can have potentially serious side effects, such as damage to the liver — the organ that breaks the drug down. You may be better off, at least once in awhile, to steer away from acetaminophen and take ibuprofen or another pain medication instead.

  Don't consume *any* alcohol at all when you're taking Tylenol (including any form of Tylenol, whether it's over-the-counter Tylenol or prescribed medications with Tylenol in them like Tylenol 3, which is Tylenol and codeine). When Tylenol is combined with alcohol, it can cause a severe liver toxicity, which means serious damage to your liver. Livers come only one to a customer, and you can't live without your liver. So take good care of it, and be extremely careful about your alcohol/Tylenol consumption. The best way to do that is to not drink when taking Tylenol.

- **Aspirin:** Aspirin can be a very effective painkiller, and it's also often used (usually at very low daily doses) by people who are at risk of suffering from heart attacks or strokes or from having another stroke.

  But aspirin can also cause serious gastrointestinal upset, and it may even lead to stomach bleeding as well as the development of *gastritis*, an inflammation of the stomach. Don't assume that aspirin is always "safe" just because you've been taking it all your life. It's still a drug. Use aspirin with caution.

- **Ibuprofen:** Ibuprofen is the generic name for Motrin or other forms of the drug. It's a painkilling drug that's available over the counter. The primary benefit of ibuprofen is the pain relief that it can bring.

  The main drawback is that it can cause serious gastrointestinal distress, including ulcers, gastritis, gastrointestinal bleeding, and so forth.

  Other possible side effects that may occur with taking ibuprofen include headaches, tinnitus (ringing in the ears), and dizziness. These side effects usually don't occur unless the patient takes high doses of the drug over a long period, but some people are more sensitive than others and may develop problems sooner.

Noting NSAIDs

Many people with fibromyalgia take OTC doses of nonsteroidal anti-inflammatory drugs, such as Aleve (generic name: naproxen sodium). This drug can often help to relieve pain; however, as with ibuprofen and other drugs, its continued use can lead to gastrointestinal disorders, such as ulcers, gastritis, and diarrhea. NSAIDS may also cause dizziness, headache, and tinnitus.

Warming up to Cold Remedies for FMS

Fibromyalgia is very different from the common cold, unless you want to factor in the generalized aches and pains of a severe flu into your "cold" equation. (Many people say that fibromyalgia feels like a semipermanent case of the flu to them, with periodic breaks of feeling a little better.)

Despite this difference, some remedies that are given to people with colds, bronchitis, and related ailments may be helpful to people who have fibromyalgia. I cover guaifenesin (a remedy that's effective in coping with cough) at the beginning of the chapter, so I'll move on to other cold remedies that people with FMS have tried.

Dealing with dextromethorphan

Some studies have researched whether taking regular doses of *dextromethorphan,* an anticough medication, could help some people cope more effectively with their symptoms of fibromyalgia. Some researchers who've studied dextromethorphan, such as Dr. Bennett, a prominent rheumatologist, initially found that low levels of dextromethorphan were ineffective in subjects with fibromyalgia. However, when the dosage of dextromethorphan was increased, their research subjects reported that their pain had significantly decreased.

In one study of the effectiveness of dextromethorphan, the drug was found to *potentiate,* or boost the effect of Ultram (generic name: tramadol), a prescribed painkilling medication. But further studies are needed before I can recommend dextromethorphan as an OTC remedy for fibromyalgia.

Some people don't want to wait, though, and they're already trying dextromethorphan now. People who follow this course should discuss it first with their physicians to make sure that taking dextromethorphan won't interact with any other medications that they take and will be safe for them.

Locating a source for dextromethorphan tablets as a stand-alone drug may be difficult because it's usually an ingredient in cold medicines. You can ask your pharmacist to order it for you in the OTC strength. (Obviously, the pharmacist won't give you the prescribed strength without a prescription from your doctor.)

Another possible option is to purchase Delsym (generic name: dextromethorphan polistirex). This OTC drug comes in a liquid form, and supposedly, it's chemically akin to dextromethorphan. (Delsym does include a small amount of alcohol, and thus, may be sedating.)

Trying antihistamines

In addition to cough medicine, some other drugs that are normally classified as *antihistamines*, or "cold medicines" may give some people with fibromyalgia some (or even a lot of) relief from their overall aches and pains. The most popular examples are Benadryl and Tylenol PM.

Cold or allergy medications may help some people with fibromyalgia because they may affect the serotonin levels, much as some antidepressants also can alleviate some of the pain and other symptoms of fibromyalgia by affecting the circulating levels of neurochemicals.

Because many antihistamines can make you drowsy, they may also help with sleep problems. But be careful with driving or any activities that require alertness when you take these drugs, unless they specify that they're "non-drowsy."

Talking About Topical Remedies

Can you really gain any pain relief from using an over-the-counter ointment that you (or a designated rubber) merely rub into your skin? Sometimes they *can* help you, even if the relief lasts only a few hours, at best. Often these drugs are listed as helpful for people with arthritis, but they can be beneficial for people with fibromyalgia too.

Considering your options

These skin ointments are available in any pharmacy and most supermarkets, and there are too many brands to list here. Most of them are creams, but there are a few spray-on remedies. Most of them contain minor anesthetics such as the following ingredients:

- **Capsaicin (derived from chili peppers):** When it works, capsaicin can actually anesthetize the parts of your body where you've rubbed it into your skin by reducing your level of Substance P (the pain neuro-chemical) and also by dulling the pain receptors at the level of your skin's surface.

- **Cayenne (comes from hot peppers):** Like capsaicin, cayenne is a substance that can cause the skin to heat up, thus causing the muscles to relax.

- **Eucalyptus (taken from the tree that is the major diet of koala bears):** This substance can act as a mild stimulant to the skin, causing tense muscles to loosen up.

- **Menthol:** You may find that menthol "cleans out your sinuses" with its very pronounced aroma. It may also provide you with temporary relief from your minor muscle pains and strains.

- **Methyl salicylate (derived from aspirin):** Many topical ointments include salicylate, which is an aspirin-based substance. These drugs may act as *both* a combination painkiller and an anesthetic when they're rubbed into the skin. They also have the benefit of bypassing the gastrointestinal system altogether, so if you've found that aspirin usually hurts your stomach, that won't likely be a problem for you with a skin rub.

- **Peppermint oil:** Often thought of solely as a flavoring, peppermint oil can also be a mild painkiller to sore and tense muscles. Don't eat your topical cream, however, or make a mint julep out of it. Very bad (and dangerous) idea.

In addition to these ointments, a variety of other ingredients can help to numb muscle pain that's close to the surface of the skin. (Your doctor can also recommend prescribed topical agents. They may include the same types of ingredients, but at a significantly greater strength.)

When you or anyone else uses a topical ointment, make sure that the person who's doing the rubbing thoroughly washes their hands directly afterwards. You don't want this substance to be inadvertently and accidentally applied to your eyes or to anyone else's, or to any other body part that may be sensitive to burning.

Deciding which topical remedy is best

One of the main difficulties with topical remedies lies in choosing which one to buy! You've got so many different ones to choose from that you may find it really hard to decide which one's the right one for you. Don't go by price only: The cheapest ointment isn't always the best choice — nor is the most expensive ointment necessarily the most effective.

When you're looking at various brands of topical ointments to help you ease your muscular aches and pains, here are a few pointers to take into consideration before making a purchase:

- ✔ **Have you bought this particular brand before?** If it worked for you before, it may work yet again. If it didn't work before, no matter how the packaging may have changed or what new and dramatic promises are made in advertisements, it probably still won't work for you now.

- ✔ **Is this drug odor-free or will everyone within 500 yards know you're coming if you use this product?** More important, do you care? If you want to be unnoticed while out in the world, choose the drug that doesn't come with the obnoxious aroma. If it doesn't matter because you're going to bed, and you don't care what you smell like as long as you get some pain relief, skip this criterion.

- ✔ **Can you buy a small tube, or even a small "sample-sized" container of the medication, in case you haven't tried this drug before, and you don't know yet if it'll help you?** If you don't like the medication, you won't have wasted your money on the larger and pricier size. If a small or sample size isn't available, you may just have to risk the wasted money if you really think the product may work for you.

- ✔ **What are the ingredients in this medication?** Does the drug have any particular ingredients that you'd prefer to avoid? Some people want to stay away from drugs that include salicylate (aspirin) in them. Perhaps, you don't like another particular ingredient, for whatever reason. Also, be sure to check for any included ingredients that you know you're allergic to.

- ✔ **Is this drug reasonably priced, and can you afford it?** When you're in severe pain, almost any amount may seem reasonable. But don't let yourself get ripped off by people taking advantage of your desperation. Check the label for the ingredients. The expensive stuff may include virtually the same ingredients as you'd also find in the lower-cost drug.

Chapter 10:

Prescribing Health with Medications

● ●

● ●

*N*atalie has had fibromyalgia for approximately ten years, and she says that she absolutely could not get through a single day without her medication. She says that she honestly believes that she'd be suicidal from the pain by now without taking her medications. The few times Natalie's waited until the last minute to refill her prescriptions and had to go a day before she got her medicine (because the pharmacy had just run out of the drug), were not days that you'd want to be around her, Natalie says.

Is Natalie a drug addict, or maybe a hypochondriac? No, she fits neither category. Natalie isn't a drug addict because she's taking her medication to alleviate her pain and not to induce pleasure. Nor is Natalie a hypochondriac. Hypochondriacs misinterpret their symptoms and worry about imagined illnesses, but fibromyalgia pain is undeniably real, and it's also often very severe. Natalie says that the medications she takes don't take *all* the pain away; they make her pain tolerable, so she can lead a relatively normal life.

Dave also has fibromyalgia, but he takes medications intermittently. Sometimes, the pain is severe, and he needs to take a strong painkiller. Other days, he's able to forego taking any medication altogether.

You may be more like Natalie, needing to take medications daily, or maybe you're more like Dave, who doesn't need medicines every day. But when you have fibromyalgia, at some point in time, you'll need prescribed medications. The purpose of this chapter is to discuss the key drugs that doctors prescribe for fibromyalgia syndrome (FMS) and the benefits and risks associated with these drugs. I talk about muscle relaxants, painkilling medications, nonsteroidal anti-inflammatory drugs, other medications used nowadays, and drugs you may see in the future. I also discuss the current controversy among doctors about prescribing painkillers and how this controversy affects some patients with fibromyalgia. So read on and find out how you can combat the pain.

Relaxing Your FMS: Muscle Relaxants

Many people with fibromyalgia complain of muscle aches and pains, so many physicians prescribe *muscle relaxants*. These drugs do just what they sound like: They soothe your over-tensed muscles and reduce the level of muscle pain.

Be sure to avoid alcohol when you're taking any muscle relaxants. One muscle relaxant, Soma (carispodal), can cause an opium-like high in some people when it's combined with alcohol. Also, even if you *don't* drink, avoid driving when taking any muscle relaxants. The sedating effects of the muscle relaxant can cause you to become an impaired driver.

Naming names

Flexeril (generic name: cyclobenzaprine) is the most commonly prescribed muscle relaxant. This drug can also act as a mild antidepressant because Flexeril increases the level of serotonin in the bloodstream. People who take Flexeril generally take it in the evening because it can cause sleepiness. Flexeril may work well for you, or it may not. Often, the only way to know for sure is to try it and see what effect it has on your aching body. One study of 120 patients with fibromyalgia indicated that 84 percent of the patients who took Flexeril significantly improved. They experienced decreased pain, improved sleep, and a reduction in the number of their tender points.

Here are a some examples of other muscle relaxants that are often prescribed to treat FMS pain (again, they may be effective or they may not be):

- Baclofen (generic name: liorisol)
- Norflex (generic name: orphenadrine citrate).

✔ Skelaxin (generic name: metaxalone),

✔ Soma (generic name: carisoprodol),

✔ Zanaflex (generic name: tizanidine HCl)

A combination of Soma and acetaminophen is also available. It's called Soma Compound.

Weighing the risks and benefits of muscle relaxants

The primary benefits of muscle relaxants are that they may provide temporary pain relief. In addition, though, the sedating action of most muscle relaxants can help those FMS patients who have trouble sleeping to avoid yet another sleepless night.

On the negative side, the chief side effect of many muscle relaxants is *gastrointestinal distress,* such as stomach pain and diarrhea. This gastrointestinal problem may range from mild to severe, depending on the particular drug and the particular patient. At the extreme end of side effects, muscle relaxants can cause damage to the stomach, such as *gastritis* (an inflammation of the stomach) or even stomach or *duodenal* (small intestine) ulcers.

Although one drug in a class of medications may cause side effects, sometimes, another drug in the same class may not cause the same side effects. Thus, if your doctor orders another muscle relaxant even after you tried one muscle relaxant that caused side effects, you should try it because you may have better luck with another drug.

Easing Pain with Painkillers

Most people with fibromyalgia *need* to take prescribed painkilling medications, at least some of the time, in order to cope with the widespread pain and stiffness — symptoms that are so characteristic of FMS.

Of course, some people with fibromyalgia may not need to take their painkilling medications every single day. Also, on some days, muscle relaxants, milder painkillers, or even over-the-counter *analgesics* (painkillers) may be sufficient to manage the pain for many people who have fibromyalgia.

Considering key pros and cons of painkilling medications

The most obvious pro, or benefit, of taking a painkilling medication is that if it works (and it's at a high enough dose), the medication makes your pain go away or makes it more tolerable. But painkilling meds have a few other benefits as well:

- ✔ If you take a painkilling medication at the same time as your pain is continuing on its upwards path, you can often thwart the pain from getting any worse and prevent it from reaching the high scream-zone of agony. In that way, your painkilling medication is acting as a preventive medicine.

- ✔ Taking painkillers when you're in severe pain can also aid your immune system. How? Basically, your body won't need to divert so much effort and energy to concentrating so hard on coping with the pain. With pain relief, your immune system can work much more efficiently.

Taking painkilling medications also has some disadvantages that every person should consider before taking these drugs.

- ✔ Side effects may be problematic for you, causing you to feel extremely drowsy and unable to drive yourself to work, school, or anywhere else that you want to go. Painkilling drugs can also be very constipating, causing you to need to change your diet (eating more fiber, fruit, and vegetables) or to take laxatives.

- ✔ Painkilling medications may also be expensive, depending on the particular drug that's ordered. Generally, the older forms are the least expensive, and they're also most likely to be available in a generic form.

- ✔ Another problem that often arises is that your doctor may be very hesitant to prescribe painkilling medications, as many doctors are, because of state and federal laws designed to curb drug abuse. You may feel like your doctor regards you as a drug addict simply because you asked him for pain medication to give you some relief. Read more about why some doctors are hesitant to prescribe painkillers later in this chapter.

Investigating controlled/scheduled drugs

Some painkillers fall into controlled drugs categories, including narcotics. (All narcotics are controlled drugs.) The federal agency known as the Drug Enforcement Administration (DEA) has designated specific medications as *scheduled drugs* or *controlled* because they are perceived as particularly dangerous, addicting, or habit forming. Drugs that are designated as scheduled drugs require more monitoring and record keeping by doctors and pharmacists because of their high potential for abuse. Some controlled drugs are painkillers that can help people with fibromyalgia, and others are only used for abuse, such as heroin.

One group of controlled drugs that's often used to treat the pain associated with fibromyalgia is narcotics.

A *narcotic* is a painkilling drug that has been classified as having a significant risk to cause addiction. Many narcotics are opium based (such as morphine and codeine), while others are synthetically derived, such as meperidine (Demerol) and methadone. From a patient's perspective, the key benefit to a narcotic is the pain relief that it provides and the return of physical and social functioning. However, many potential side effects are possible with narcotics.

Narcotics aren't the only drugs that have been identified by the DEA as potential drugs of abuse. Amphetamines, anabolic steroids, and other types of drugs are also considered addicting drugs, and they've been "scheduled" by the DEA. (See the sidebar on scheduled drugs and FMS.) These non-narcotic drugs are generally not sedating, nor are they used for their painkilling properties, as are narcotics.

The most feared side effect is addiction, but that rarely occurs among people taking narcotics to alleviate pain rather than to attain an artificial "high." The side effects that often do occur are sedation, dry mouth, and constipation.

At very high doses, narcotics can also cause considerable mental confusion or anxiety and may even result in *hallucinations* (seeing, hearing, or feeling things that aren't really there). They may also cause *delusions* (believing things that aren't true), for example, that aliens have landed in the back yard, or the government has planted secret listening devices in newspapers.

Prescribing painkillers: The dilemma

For some people with fibromyalgia, their pain is constant and severe, and it can only be made bearable by taking painkilling medications. Some people with fibromyalgia say that their doctors are extremely resistant about prescribing any painkilling medications, telling them to take regular Tylenol or ibuprofen if they have pain. Others say that as long as the drug isn't on the scheduled drug list, their doctor will give it to them. When doctors deny FMS sufferers these medications, their severe pain continues, and they have great difficulty navigating through the daily dramas and requirements of life.

Scheduled drugs and FMS

Under the Controlled Substances Act, passed by Congress in 1970, controlled drugs — some of which are illegal — fall into five *schedules* (or categories) of drugs, based on the level of addictiveness, with Schedule I having the highest risk of addiction and Schedule V the lowest of this group:

✔ Schedule I: Drugs that have been categorized as having major potential for drug abuse. Such drugs as heroin and LSD are in Schedule I. These drugs have no value to patients who have fibromyalgia.

✔ Schedule II: These drugs also have potential for abuse, albeit somewhat less than drugs in Schedule I. Cocaine is included on the Schedule II list (some doctors have legitimate uses for the drug), as is methadone. Some fibromyalgia patients may take methadone for pain control, and others take Percocet or Percodan (both are forms of oxycodone). Some people with fibromyalgia have also used OxyContin and found it beneficial, in large part, because of its timed-release benefit. Unfortunately, OxyContin has become a very popular drug for people wanting to abuse drugs to gain a "high." As a result of this problem, legitimate patients are having a hard time receiving prescriptions for OxyContin.

✔ Schedule III: This category includes medications, such as Tylenol 3 (Tylenol with codeine) Vicodin (a form of hydrocodone), and barbiturate medications, such as Fiorcet (butalbital). Some fibromyalgia patients take these drugs for pain control.

✔ Schedule IV: Patients with fibromyalgia needing an anti-anxiety drug may take Valium (generic name: diazepam) or Xanax (generic name: alprazolam), which both fall under this schedule.

✔ Schedule V: Some medications that include codeine, such as cough syrups with codeine, are categorized by the DEA as scheduled drugs. These drugs are generally less helpful for people with fibromyalgia.

Judy says that she could probably score cocaine easier than she could convince her doctor to give her a prescription for Ultram (generic name: tramadol), a mild *analgesic* (painkiller) that's not even on the controlled drug list. And she says that she knows she can totally forget about ever asking her doctor for a controlled drug. She tried once, and after she asked him, Judy says that the look of horror on his face made it very clear where he stood in terms of prescribing narcotic painkillers.

Many people with fibromyalgia find it degrading to have to beg their doctor for painkillers. Even worse, if a doctor reluctantly provides a small number of painkillers, the contrast between the relatively pain-free existence and the return of the pain when the limited supply of pills is gone is maddening.

Tom says that he receives prescriptions for narcotics from his doctor that he can take when the pain becomes very bad to intolerable, but his physician also keeps a very close watch on his dosage and asks Tom plenty of questions, such as where the pain is, how bad it is, and so forth. Tom is very careful about taking strong drugs, and he uses them only for severe pain. Otherwise, he relies on milder medications. Tom feels that his doctor has just the right balance of compassion combined with careful control.

Painkillers, particularly narcotics and other controlled drugs, are not drugs to take lightly, and any doctor who does so isn't the physician for you.

But in my experience the problem usually isn't a doctor who dispenses painkillers freely, but it's rather that some doctors are resistant to prescribing painkilling medications. Why are doctors often reluctant to prescribe strong painkillers for relief of fibromyalgia-related pain?

- ✔ Doctors disagree on whether narcotics are effective at treating the pain of fibromyalgia. Many doctors think that narcotics are usually ineffective; others think that they can relieve at least some of the severe pain.

- ✔ The side effects associated with narcotic painkillers are of concern to many doctors. (See the "Investigating controlled/scheduled drugs" section earlier in this chapter.)

- ✔ Few doctors want to be regarded as "easy" when it comes to writing prescriptions for strong painkilling medications. They risk their professional careers, if tagged with such a label.

- ✔ Many doctors are afraid of having to deal with law enforcement agencies. Law enforcement agencies in many states have become concerned about the abuse of prescription medications, particularly of controlled drugs. Drug abusers don't take controlled drugs for pain control. They take them to attain an artificial high, or they take them because they've become addicted to the drug (often because the drugs were originally taken to get high). Sometimes, people who are in severe pain also become addicted to painkillers, if their physicians give them very high doses and are otherwise careless.

  Drug abusers develop such an overwhelming need for the drug that they will forge prescriptions, steal drugs from pharmacies, or buy them on the street. These people are the ones that law enforcement agencies are concerned about.

Unfortunately, some patients who have severe pain are the victims of overzealous law enforcement and frightened physicians. The drug addicts and the people who seek illegal highs will find their drugs somewhere. The hurting patients who need legitimate pain relief don't have that alternative, unless they're willing to acquire the medications illegally.

Fighting pain with non-narcotic pills

Ultram (generic name: tramadol) is a non-narcotic drug (not under the Controlled Substances Act or overseen by the Drug Enforcement Administration) that's effective at alleviating pain for many people with fibromyalgia. A more recent variation of Ultram is *Ultracet*, which is a medication that combines Ultram with Tylenol (acetaminophen). It's not clear to researchers exactly how these drugs work, but they appear to work similarly to a narcotic drug in inhibiting pain, although in a milder and less dangerous way.

So what can you do if you're in pain, but your doctor seems (or definitely is) hesitant to prescribe narcotic painkilling medication? You can use several tactics. First, you can ask your doctor bluntly if she's concerned that you'll become addicted to medication. Whether she says yes or no, you can point out that you've never developed an addiction in the past. (If that's true.) Next, you can state that you're seeking medication to combat pain, not to go off on some sort of high.

Finally, it's always a good idea to give one or two examples of what your pain is preventing you from doing. Maybe you can't drive your children to soccer practice anymore, even though it's really important to you, because you're hurting so bad. Or perhaps you feel like a prisoner in your house because the pain is so overwhelming. If your candor and your examples don't seem to matter, and your doctor can't or won't give you a reason that makes sense to you for why she won't prescribe a painkiller, it's probably time for you to read Chapter 7, my chapter on how to find a new physician.

Reducing Inflammation: NSAIDs

Some individuals with fibromyalgia obtain significant pain relief by taking prescribed (or over-the-counter) doses of *nonsteroidal anti-inflammatory drugs* (NSAIDs). The most commonly used drugs in this category are Naprosyn (generic name: naproxen sodium), Feldene (generic name: piroxicam), Motrin (ibuprofen), and Relafen (generic name: nabumetone). Some patients with fibromyalgia have also benefited from the most recently introduced NSAIDs — Vioxx (generic name: rofecoxib), Celebrex (generic name: celecoxib), and Bextra (generic name: valdecoxib). Bextra is the new kid on the block when it comes to NSAID drugs, as of this writing. The FDA approved it in late 2001. These newer drugs seem to have less serious side effects than the older NSAIDs.

Vioxx and Bextra have the capability to reduce pain as well as stiffness and inflammation, and when you have fibromyalgia, a drug that can attack all these problems is certainly worthy of consideration. However, individuals who are allergic to sulfa drugs (such as the antibiotic Septra) should not take Celebrex.

NSAIDs generally are taken by fibromyalgia sufferers on a daily basis to combat chronic pain, and they can be moderately effective. The primary drawback to NSAID medications is that they can cause gastrointestinal upset, which can sometimes be severe. For this reason, they should always be taken with meals, and NSAIDs should never be taken on an empty stomach. In some cases, NSAIDs can cause ulcers. Anyone who's experiencing severe abdominal pain should stop taking their NSAID medication immediately and should consult with their physician. Other side effects may include rashes, rapid heartbeat, stuffy nose, blurred vision, and lightheadedness.

Some people take over-the-counter medications, such as Tums or Rolaids, along with their NSAID medication, to prevent stomach upset. Others make sure that they only take the medication with food, and that action alone is enough to alleviate the gastrointestinal distress that would occur if they took the medication on an empty stomach. Newer forms of NSAIDS, a class known as "COX-2 inhibitors," are less likely to cause gastrointestinal problems. They're designed to be gentler on your stomach. However, some individuals who take these medications may still develop gastrointestinal symptoms.

Many physicians recommend that these newer drugs should be taken with meals, even though you may not be given these instructions on your prescription bottle, as you usually would with other prescribed NSAIDs. (Doctors like to be extra careful.)

Fighting FMS with Antidepressants

Many people with fibromyalgia take one or more antidepressant medications. These medications include:

- ✔ Adapin (generic name: doxepin)
- ✔ Desyrel (generic name: trazodone)
- ✔ Effexor (generic name: venlafaxine)
- ✔ Elavil (generic name: amitriptyline)

- Pamelor (generic name: nortriptyline)

- Paxil (generic name: paroxetine)

- Prozac (generic name: fluoxetine)

- Serzone (generic name: nefazodone)

- Zoloft (generic name: sertraline)

Two of the more common antidepressant medications used by people with FMS are Elavil and Prozac.

I'm not depressed! Why do I need an antidepressant?

Some patients with fibromyalgia *may* have a problem with depression. But, often, people with fibromyalgia are taking antidepressants not for depression, but rather for their fibromyalgia. Research has demonstrated that low doses of some antidepressants, taken on a daily basis (or, rather, nightly because most doctors recommend the drugs be taken in the evening), can help block the pain of fibromyalgia or other chronic pain.

You may be worried about the advisability of taking a "psychiatric" drug for a condition that you don't have. However, most doctors agree that the very low doses of antidepressants that are prescribed to provide pain control for patients with fibromyalgia (and who have other chronic medical problems) aren't high enough to be sufficiently effective at treating true depression. The point is, the doses of antidepressants that are prescribed to treat fibromyalgia are usually so low that, even if you *were* depressed, you wouldn't gain any relief from your depression at those low levels of medication. (Read more about fibromyalgia and depression in Chapter 16.)

Sometimes, doctors will prescribe two antidepressants at the same time for their patients with fibromyalgia, hoping they'll gain increased relief. For example, in one clinical study, fibromyalgia patients were given both Elavil (25 mgs.) and Prozac (20 mgs.). The result: a significant number of patients actually received twice the pain relief with this combination than they gained with either drug by itself. Although you may intuitively think that taking two drugs *would* logically give you about twice the relief as you'd receive from taking one medication, in actuality, that effect rarely happens. As a result, if and when research shows such significant pain control, this fact makes researchers stand up and pay attention. Of course, no one should take two different antidepressants unless their doctor recommends it.

Thinking about pluses and minuses of antidepressants

The good news about using antidepressants to treat fibromyalgia pain is that many antidepressants are relatively inexpensive, and most doctors will not hesitate to prescribe these medications for the treatment of chronic pain problems. In other words, you generally don't need to see a psychiatrist in order to receive a prescription for an antidepressant.

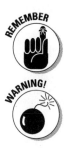

However, if you or your doctor think that you *might* actually have a severe form of depression, you're really better off consulting with a psychiatrist. Why? Psychiatrists are the most knowledgeable physicians when it comes to antidepressants and other drugs that help people who have emotional problems.

As with all medications, antidepressants have potential side effects:

- ✔ Constipation
- ✔ Diminished libido (lowered sex drive) or complete lack of libido

  When that effect occurs, it usually goes away when the drug is out of the system, and normal libido will return.
- ✔ Headaches or a "druggy" feeling
- ✔ Insomnia
- ✔ Upset stomach
- ✔ Weight gain or weight loss

Often (although not always), the initial side effects decrease or go away completely after the person's body becomes more accustomed to the drug.

Other Prescribed Medicines for FMS

A variety of other categories of drugs may also be very helpful in treating the symptoms of fibromyalgia, particularly the symptom that probably bothers you the most — the pain. Doctors may prescribe anti-epileptic (also known as anticonvulsant) drugs, anti-anxiety drugs, and antihistamines for pain relief.

Talking about trigger-point injections

When your pain is severe and seems to be isolated to one or several clearly defined areas, some physicians consider using treatments of trigger-point injections. These injections are usually given directly into or nearby the zones where the pain dominates. Often, patients with fibromyalgia suffer from the trigger points of *myofascial pain syndrome,* another pain syndrome that's discussed in Chapter 6. These trigger points (different from tender points) are painful ropey areas that the physician can actually feel during an examination.

Most doctors inject 1-percent procaine or lidocaine into the area that's the most painful. These injections can be given several times per year, and many patients with fibromyalgia gain considerable pain relief from them. The injections are usually given on an outpatient basis, and they have only minor side effects, such as slight bruising. If you experience any pain at the injection site, icing or heating the area usually provides relief. Some people may have an allergic reaction to lidocaine injections, however.

The physician who injects the medication should be a neurologist, anesthesiologist, or rheumatologist because these types of specialists usually have the most experience with treating both fibromyalgia and pain. An inexperienced physician may perform too many injections, or inject medications into the wrong areas.

Evaluating anti-epileptic drugs

Some physicians prescribe anti-epileptic drugs for purposes of pain relief for their FMS patients even if those patients have never had a seizure in their lives. Anti-epileptics can calm hyperactive pain fibers. The only way to know for sure whether such a drug works is to take the medication and note its effects on you. The key side effects that these drugs have are that they may be very sedating, and they may also cause dry mouth and dizziness. These drugs include such medications as Neurontin (generic name: gabapentin), Topamax (generic name: topiramate), and Lamictal (generic name: lamotrigine).

Pondering anti-anxiety medicines

Sometimes, anti-anxiety drugs can alleviate some symptoms of fibromyalgia. Anxiety makes pain worse, and thus decreasing anxiety can be very helpful in pain control. If the drugs work, the individual has relief from some symptoms of fibromyalgia, such as problems with sleeping. The drugs can also induce a level of calmness to combat the high stress that most people suffering from fibromyalgia experience.

Some anti-anxiety drugs are Valium (generic name: diazepam) or Xanax (generic name: alprazolam). Both of these are scheduled/controlled drugs by the Drug Enforcement Administration, because of their potential for addiction.

Some physicians may prescribe Klonopin (generic name: clonazepam). Sometimes, the drug Restoril (generic name: temazepam) is prescribed for patients with fibromyalgia. Other physicians may prescribe the antidepressants Paxil or Prozac as anti-anxiety medications.

Generally, lower doses of anti-anxiety drugs are used to treat fibromyalgia. However, some people with fibromyalgia need higher doses of anti-anxiety drugs than would be indicated for treating fibromyalgia alone because they actually do suffer from both fibromyalgia and anxiety. (See Chapter 16 for more information on emotional problems, such as anxiety and depression, among people with fibromyalgia.)

Anti-anxiety drugs can be highly sedating, and they may also cause nightmares. Other side effects of these medications are dizziness and lightheadedness. Of even greater concern, some anti-anxiety drugs may be habit forming, particularly Xanax (generic name: alprazolam). As a result, they have the potential to become addicting if not taken properly. (*Habit-forming* is a lower level of *addiction*.)

Don't take these drugs when you need to drive or operate equipment. Also, keep in mind the fact that after you start taking one of these medications, you shouldn't stop them without consulting with your physician. The reason: If a person who's used to taking the drug suddenly stops taking it, he or she may suffer from convulsions or other serious withdrawal effects.

Analyzing antihistamines

Although further research must be done, a few studies have indicated that some antihistamines have mild *analgesic* (painkilling) qualities. Histamine is a pain-promoting substance made by the body, and conversely, antihistamine counteracts histamine. For example, Atarax (generic name: hyroxyzine) provides some pain relief, and it's also mildly sedating.

Researchers in Denmark found a new antihistamine, ReN 1869, which reduced inflammation and pain in laboratory mice, with no apparent ill effects. They reported on their finding in a 2002 issue of the *European Journal of Pharmacology*. It'll be years (if ever) before such antihistamines can be used by humans. Still, such research is encouraging.

Opening Your Eyes to Info on Sleep Remedies

If dark circles under your eyes and severe tiredness due to lack of sleep accompany your other symptoms of fibromyalgia, you're definitely not alone. Most people with fibromyalgia have severe sleep problems. If you're deprived of the restorative qualities of a good night's sleep and the opportunity for your body to rest and recuperate from the day's ordeals, this lack of sleep can greatly worsen your symptoms of pain, muscle stiffness, and fatigue.

You can choose from many ways to cope with your sleep deficit, such as using relaxation therapy or hypnosis or avoiding certain foods. (Read Chapter 14 for more information on sleep and fibromyalgia, and tactics for improving your sleep.) Medications can help, too.

Many of the medications described in this chapter, such as antidepressants, muscle relaxants, and painkilling drugs, have a side effect of causing drowsiness. Some NSAIDs, prescribed for muscle pain and stiffness, may also cause some individuals to feel drowsy. But sometimes, sleep-deprived people need a drug that was specifically designed to cope with sleep problems.

Today, Ambien (generic name: zolpidem) is the primary medication that's prescribed for sleep difficulties. (Read more about Ambien in Chapter 14 on dealing with sleep problems.) Other medications that are sometimes used are Mogadon (generic name: nitrazepam) and Desyrel (generic name: trazodone), an antidepressant.

Evaluating whether sleep medication is needed

Only your doctor can decide whether a specific sleep remedy should be prescribed. However, here are some indications that a sleep remedy may be necessary:

- Sleeping less than five hours per night
- Frequently waking up at night (more than two to three times every evening)
- Severe daytime drowsiness from lack of sleep
- Apparent impairment from lack of sleep (stumbling about, frequent instances of forgetfulness, inattentiveness)

Looking at the ups and downs of sleep remedies

The most obvious benefit of a sleep remedy is that it induces or at least helps you to attain some much-needed sleep. If you're fully rested and your body has had a chance to release hormones needed by a healthy body, such as growth hormone and others, your fibromyalgia symptoms will likely improve as well.

Although sleep remedies can be a godsend for many people, they do have some downsides. Ambien, although usually harmless, can cause continued drowsiness, and diarrhea in some people. Desyrel can cause continued sleepiness and weight gain. Mogadon may be habit forming and may also cause headaches, dizziness, and loss of libido. Mogadon is only indicated for the most severe cases of insomnia.

As with all drugs, doctors should carefully consider potential side effects before prescribing a sleep remedy. They should also take into account other medications that you're already taking because, sometimes, drugs interact with each other, boosting or weakening the effect of each other or causing other reactions.

Thinking About Future Remedies

Because so many people suffer from the symptoms of fibromyalgia, pharmaceutical companies are working very hard to develop medications that are specifically effective for people with fibromyalgia. As a result, new and better treatments should be available within the next few years or even sooner. So hang on, if you're dissatisfied with the medications that are available now. Help is on its way.

As of this writing, research appears to be surging ahead on several parallel fronts.

- **Growth hormones:** Some researchers have already shown that injections of growth hormone have improved the symptoms of some patients with fibromyalgia. Further study is needed, however. The key problem with this particular therapy is that growth hormone is very expensive, and until the price comes down further, it can't be used as a therapy for fibromyalgia patients.

- **Antidepressant and anti-epileptic medications:** Promising research on these drugs is occurring at present, and this research is likely to lead to improved treatments for people with fibromyalgia.

- **Pregabalin:** One exciting medication candidate for fibromyalgia relief is pregabalin, a new antiseizure drug that's been shown to specifically improve the symptoms of fibromyalgia in several clinical trials.

- **Duloxetine:** This drug is an antidepressant medication that will soon be available for fibromyalgia pain.

✔ **Interferon:** In other research, Amarillo Biosciences, Inc., based in Amarillo, Texas, is testing the feasibility of an oral lozenge that contains *interferon-alpha,* an immunity-boosting drug. Preliminary research in two clinical trials has revealed that patients with fibromyalgia gained significant relief from morning stiffness, and research is ongoing. Preliminary research has indicated that interferon has significantly improved fibromyalgia symptoms in some patients, and larger clinical studies that are planned should provide additional information.

According to Amarillo Biosciences president and CEO Joseph Cummins, the oral lozenge that his company is currently testing contains only 50 IU (international units) of interferon-alpha, compared to the 3 million units that's usually used with injected interferon. As a result, interferon in lozenge form will be much lower priced than injected interferon. Cummins believes that nearly all patients with fibromyalgia will be able to afford his interferon lozenge.

According to Cummins, as soon as the FDA gives the thumbs-up approval to the company, the drug can become available to the public. However, performing clinical studies and gaining FDA approval for a new medication takes plenty of time and money, and Cummins says that, if approved, 2005 is probably about the earliest that his company's interferon lozenges could become available to people with fibromyalgia.

I really can't say exactly when drugs that are currently in the "pipeline" (in clinical testing) as of this writing will actually receive FDA approval and become available to fibromyalgia patients down the road. Medications can't be prescribed for patients until they've been both thoroughly tested in clinical trials and approved by the FDA to be sold to patients in the U.S. But probably within the next two to five years, FMS sufferers will have many new choices to treat the pain, fatigue, and other symptoms of fibromyalgia.

Chapter 11

Using Hands-On Therapies

. . . .

. . . .

*W*hen you're suffering from major pain, even the thought of a little hands-on therapy can make you cringe or shudder. Nobody likes to be touched when his or her body hurts, especially in those places *where* the body's really hurting.

But sometimes, hands-on therapy can really help, whether the touching comes from cold therapy, heat therapy, massage therapy, or, in some cases, from special machines that act to stimulate and relax the tender areas.

In this chapter, I provide basic information about these hands-on techniques, including how they work, why they work, what to watch out for, and how these different options may just help you reduce the pain of your fibromyalgia syndrome (FMS).

Chilling Out! Icing the Pain

You don't have to go off and live with the penguins to obtain some ice-cold pain relief. *Cryotherapy* (also known as "cold therapy") uses cold to dull or weaken your agitated nerve endings in the area being iced, making it harder for the pain signals to reach your brain. Cryotherapy also slows the blood flow to the affected area, decreasing inflammation and pain.

Gelling the pain

You can purchase *gel packs,* which are plastic containers that are filled with a gelatinous substance. They can be frozen and applied to the painful area. Some gel packs are also enclosed in cloth. They come in many different sizes as well as a broad range of prices. You can purchase these gel packs in pharmacies or department stores, or you can buy them from companies who sell products over the Internet, at sites such as www.egeneralmedical.com/homarmit.

Gel packs may be as inexpensive as $10 each or less, and they're generally reusable. Some gel packs are designed for freezing only, but others may be frozen or heated up in your microwave oven, so that they can be used for dual therapy. Use these packs for cold therapy or heat therapy, depending on your needs.

Cryotherapy can be as close to you as your very own kitchen. Frozen water that comes from your freezer (otherwise known by its technical term *ice*) can work very well, indeed, for your personal cold therapy. Fancy ice packs and simple plastic bags that are filled with ice cubes can both do the job. Another option is to use a plastic package of frozen vegetables, straight from your freezer.

Be sure that you place a clean wash cloth or towel over your sore area and then place the ice over that. Avoid directly icing the painful area because you risk causing damage to the skin if you do. You don't want to add frostbite to your list of symptoms resulting from your fibromyalgia.

Don't leave ice packs on for any longer than about 20 to 30 minutes at a time, or you can harm your skin (even when you use the towel). Set your timer or keep your eye on your watch, and play it safe.

If you want something more advanced than a bag of frozen peas, you can make your own ice applicator very easily and inexpensively. Simply fill a paper cup with water (about ¾ full because ice expands) and then freeze it. When you want to use cryotherapy, just peel down the sides of the top of the cup and then use the rest of the cup as your applicator — similar to the way that you use a roll-on deodorant.

The pain relief from cold therapy is usually temporary, lasting several hours at most. However, when you're in severe pain from a flare-up of your fibromyalgia, even a mere few hours of relief is a worthwhile goal, indeed.

If you suffer from frequent headaches, as many people with fibromyalgia do, try this simple remedy: Place an ice pack on the back of your neck for about 20 minutes. This cold can often help block the pain pathway, confusing the neurochemical pain messengers. Most important, it may relieve your headache.

Heating Up the Problem: Heat Therapy

Ice therapy isn't always the best way to relieve your fibromyalgia pain and muscle stiffness. The direct opposite — heat therapy — may work much more effectively for you when you're in pain and need some relief *right now*.

Heat helps by getting your blood flowing to the painful area and by speeding up the healing process. Heat relaxes stiff muscles and improves circulation, thus easing your pain. As a result, heat that's applied to the painful area may be effective in decreasing (although probably not entirely eliminating) your underlying pain.

Heat is most often best for chronic pain, such as is usually experienced by people with FMS; cold seems to work better for acute pain and inflammation. So if you're experiencing chronic pain, try heat first. But if it doesn't work for you, try cold next.

Carole, who's had fibromyalgia for ten years, says that two things — hot baths and massage therapy — have really given her significant relief from her fibromyalgia symptoms.

Delivering the heat

Even something as simple as a hot bath or shower or lying down on an inexpensive heating pad (turned to the *low* or the *medium* setting) may provide you with a major pain decrease.

Dry heat (such as a heating pad or a hot but dry towel for example) or wet heat (a hot and wet cloth or steam heat) — which is better? Sometimes, dry heat may be the best answer for you, and at other times, moist heat (using hot, wet towels or standing in a steamy shower) may ease your pain more effectively. Predicting which method, wet or dry heat, will work better for you can be hard, and, sometimes, you may need to try one and then, if it's not working, go ahead and try the other.

Some gel packs can be heated in the microwave oven and then applied to the skin. Be sure to carefully read the instructions on any such product that you buy. You may be the kind of person who hates reading instruction manuals —

many people are. But force yourself to read the basic information anyway, and don't risk experimenting on yourself. (If you don't you could get the pack too hot and burn yourself, or the pack could explode if left in the microwave too long!)

Being cautious about hot tubs

Because warmth can make you feel better, why not soak in a hot tub or spa? This choice can be a questionable one for people with fibromyalgia because the water is often uncomfortably hot (although it should never be hotter than 104° F) and can exacerbate your symptoms. But worse than that, soaking in a hot tub (especially for an extended period) can have a dangerously sedating effect, particularly when you're taking pain medications, sleep remedies, or other drugs. Some people have actually drowned in their own hot tubs when they decided to soak alone.

If you do decide to use a hot tub, make sure that the temperature is set at a tolerable level before you enter the tub. Be sure to enter the tub slowly. You don't want to leap into hot water any more than you'd want to plunge your whole hand into a boiling pot that's on your stove. Limit the amount of time that you remain in the tub to no more than 15 minutes. Also, be sure that someone else is at home with you when you use the hot tub — preferably, *in* the tub with you.

Avoiding overheating

Be sure that you don't overheat the painful areas of your body. *No pain, no gain* is an old saying that absolutely does *not* apply to fibromyalgia. The heat may be mildly discomforting, at most, but it shouldn't be painfully burning.

Second or third degree burns won't help your condition (duh). But even if the item that you're using doesn't get to that level of heat, excessive heat can result in a serious flare-up in your fibromyalgia symptoms and your pain. Avoid it.

If you're using a heating pad, it almost certainly has a temperature control. Use it. Set it to a low or medium setting. If no temperature control's available because you're using hot towels that you may have boiled or that came straight from the dryer, test the temperature by touching it quickly. If your first response when you touch the hot towel is to spring back with an "Ouch!", it's too hot for you.

Let the hot item cool down a little bit more before you think about applying it to your body. And then test it again with your hand before you lie on the hot towel or heating pad. This therapy isn't called "burning therapy," after all.

Getting down and dirty with mud baths

It may remind you of making mud pies in preschool or kindergarten, but sitting in a hot mud bath can provide you with some relief from your fibromyalgia symptoms. A 1999 study performed in Italy indicated that mud baths, combined with antidepressants, gave subjects significant relief from their symptoms of fibromyalgia.

Further study is needed before scientists will know for sure if mud baths are a valid treatment for the symptoms of fibromyalgia.

But don't tell that to Mandy, a long-time sufferer of FMS. She already knows the answer for her and says that she feels really great after her mud bath, which she receives in a spa every few weeks.

Basically, she soaks in a hot tub of peat moss for about 20 minutes, after which she gets cleaned up and rests for about a half an hour so that she'll be alert enough to drive home. Relief often lasts for days, although Mandy can't afford mud bath treatments more frequently than biweekly, because they cost $60 a shot. (Prices vary from spa to spa.)

Mud baths and sulfur bath therapy are much more popular in Europe than in the United States, so finding a place that provides such a therapy for you may be tough. Generally, spas that offer mud baths in the United States are located on the West Coast, particularly in California.

Massaging the Problem: Massage Therapy

A mild massaging of your aching muscles and other tender areas of your body can be helpful, whether the massage is performed by a professional massage therapist or by your loving partner or a friend. (A professional is preferable, if you can afford it or, even better, if your health insurance covers it.)

If no one's available to provide you with a massage, you may choose to use a mechanical massager. Be sure to set such devices to the low or the medium settings to start with. The high cycle may be far too vigorous for a person with fibromyalgia. And read the instructions on the device before you apply it to your body.

Sometimes, either heat or cold therapy is combined with massage therapy in an attempt to amplify the relief that's provided. For example, you may lie on a heating pad while the massage is being provided. Or you can take a hot bath at home and have your partner provide you with a gentle massage afterwards.

Realizing that it's not a cure, but it can be helpful

A gentle to medium massage treatment can't cure you of your fibromyalgia, but it may ease your pain for a few hours or even a day or so. When it works, massage can stimulate the production of *endorphins*, natural pain chemicals that travel to the hurting parts of your body and provide relief — somewhat like soldiers in the cavalry, rushing in to help the besieged troops at the fort. But these endorphins only stay in the bloodstream for so long. Massage therapy clearly can be very useful for some people who have fibromyalgia, but it's a therapy that needs to be repeated on a regular basis in order to continue the benefit.

A study of the effects of massage on the painful areas of people with FMS (reported in a 1999 issue of the *European Journal of Pain*) revealed that subjects who received 15 massage sessions over the course of ten weeks received significant pain relief. In fact, the 23 people in the treatment group who received massage therapy were able to reduce their use of painkilling medications.

However, the improvement for the fibromyalgia subjects who felt better from massage was only a temporary reprieve, and six months after the treatments ended, most of the pain had returned again.

Diana is a long-term fibromyalgia sufferer, and she's also a major massage therapy fan. She says that massage has been such a godsend in keeping her from completely stiffening up.

Not everyone feels so positively about massage and its value. Lauren, another person who's had FMS for years, says that massage therapy has helped her somewhat, but she also warns that massage is extremely short-term help. She says that she'd really need to *live* with a massage therapist in order for it to be both affordable and realistic for her. Because that's obviously not practical, she's foregoing massage therapy.

Not everyone can tolerate massage therapy, even when it's gentle. Louise, who has had FMS for several years, works part-time as a massage therapist herself, but she says that massage has actually made her fibromyalgia much worse. Louise has completely given up on this form of therapy for herself. She knows that massage therapy helps some people a great deal, but for her, it just doesn't work.

Working with the insurance company

Increasing numbers of health insurance companies are providing coverage for massage therapy, although the numbers of allowed visits may be limited to fewer appointments than most patients would like.

In some areas of the country, however, massage therapy is considered an important or even required therapy. For example, in the state of Washington, health insurance companies are actually required by state law to cover massage therapy for their insured individuals.

Ask your doctor if she thinks that getting a prescription for massage therapy can help you obtain health insurance coverage, or call the insurance company yourself and ask them whether they'd cover the treatment if your doctor orders it.

If you receive a *no* or if the person at the insurance company says that she's not really sure about whether coverage will be provided (with or without a prescription from your doctor), you need to decide if you're willing to open up your own purse to pay for your treatment.

Even if you decide that massage therapy is worth the money you'll have to pay, when the insurance company has said either *no* or *maybe,* consider asking your doctor to go ahead and write you a prescription for the massage therapy anyway. Then submit the prescription order with an insurance claim to your insurance company, or have the massage therapist submit it if their office handles insurance claims.

You may receive a denial of your claim in the mail. But you may also be pleasantly surprised and receive a check to reimburse you for all, or some part of, your massage therapy expenses.

Be sure that you also photocopy the prescription for the massage, so that you have backup information in case the insurance company has a question or if they lose what you've sent them. If the insurance company denies your claim, consider appealing the denial. In your appeal later, be sure to state that you have a diagnosed medical problem and that massage therapy is an important part of your treatment.

Of course, be reasonable in your expectations. You probably won't be covered by your insurance company for having daily massage therapy, even in the unlikely event that your doctor agrees that you need it that frequently. Some insurers may consider several times a week a reasonable therapy.

No shoes, no shirt, service

Don't assume that you'll need to go totally naked in order to receive massage therapy, although if you're having a full-body massage, you may need to strip down. Your body will be draped, and only the part that the therapist is working on will be uncovered. In most cases, the uncovered area doesn't include any erogenous zones, such as women's breasts or the genitals of men or women. Instead, you usually keep on your underwear, and the areas not being massaged (such as your upper or lower torso) are covered with a sheet or a towel. If the therapist tells you that you *must* strip and you don't want to, simply refuse. You may have inadvertently stumbled into the wrong type of massage facility.

Forming a non-aggression pact with your massage therapist

Be sure to make it very clear to anyone who massages your muscles — whether that person is your partner, a friend, or a trained massage therapist or physical therapist — that they must take it slower and easier with you than they normally would with people who don't have fibromyalgia. You absolutely don't want an aggressive form of massage therapy.

The reason: When people with FMS receive a very active and painful massage, that massage can be a self-defeating experience that results in a flare-up of pain. You may end up feeling much worse when you leave than you did when you came in.

If the therapist can't comply with your request for a gentle massage or simply won't listen to your firm assertion about massage and fibromyalgia that less is really more, ask the facility for another person to provide your massage. Or you may want to just "vote with your feet" and go someplace else.

If your therapist asks you whether you want the Swedish massage or the deep-tissue massage, choose the Swedish one because that's the gentle massage option.

If the massage therapist tells you that the massage may result in a little bruising, do not proceed! Any massage that causes tissue damage is a very bad idea for a person with fibromyalgia. (And not such a great idea for a person who doesn't have FMS.)

Never allow anyone to walk on your back. Doing so can cause serious damage as well as long-lasting pain.

If your partner provides the massage

Suppose that you can't afford to hire a professional massage therapist, or you just don't want to for some reason. But you do have your very own loving partner who's ready and willing to give you a back rub or to massage other sore parts. Should you let him or her provide you with a much-needed massage, even if your partner has no training? That question is really up to you.

If you decide that the answer is *yes,* follow some simple guidelines, provided below. Also remember that an adult should perform the massaging. Don't expect your child or teenager to give you regular massages. Placing your children in such an adult role is unfair to them and to you.

First, be sure to tell your partner before any massaging starts that a little discomfort is normal when painful areas are probed. But if it really hurts, it's time to immediately cease and desist with massaging that body part.

Next, realize that if the massage is being performed by your sexual partner, your partner possibly may become sexually stimulated by massaging you, even though it's your neck or your back, not any erogenous zones — and even though the last thing you feel like doing right now is having sex. (And no, a professional massage therapist whom you're not in a relationship with should *not* become aroused during a massage, in case you're wondering.)

As a result, if you're in no mood for romance and just want a gentle massage of your aching body, warn your partner ahead of time that this massage is going to be strictly business and no fooling around should be anticipated. You may want to forego the fancy scented oils altogether and, instead, go for a smelly topical lotion!

Tell your partner to keep the massage brief. He or she will probably tire fairly quickly anyway, but try to go for 15 to 20 minutes max.

Advise your partner that he or she should provide a light and nonbruising massage. The key is "nonpainful."

If your partner massages your body with electric devices, tell him or her to be cautious. Always start on the low end of the machine's capabilities. You probably won't be able to tolerate the high levels, and the experience can also make you feel worse.

Finding a massage therapist

Interested in finding a good massage therapist, but you're not quite sure where to begin to look for one? You can try starting with the yellow pages of your local phone book, but that's usually not the best place to begin your search. Why not? Because such a cursory search can't give you the opportunity for some preliminary screening options, like the kind you'll get when you ask your doctor, friends, and others for recommendations. Also, the therapist with the biggest advertisement in the phone book isn't necessarily the best one — although he may be.

Asking around

Here are a few ideas to get you started in identifying a good massage therapist:

- ✔ Ask your physician if he can recommend anyone who performs massage therapy, or if he knows anyone else who may be able to recommend someone. Also, ask your doctor's nurses if they know of anyone who performs massage therapy.

- ✔ Ask your friends and coworkers if they can recommend a massage therapist (but also know that you'll probably receive a little — or maybe a lot of — teasing).

- ✔ Contact fitness centers in the area. (Often, members who are into exercising big time also enjoy receiving massages for their aching muscles.)

Another way to locate a massage therapist in your own back yard is to contact the *American Massage Therapy Association,* a national organization of therapists. If you live in the United States, you can call them toll-free at 888-843-2682. If you're not a U.S. resident or simply prefer the Internet, you can go to their Web site (www.amtamassage.org) to search for a local massage therapist.

Screening the therapist

After you find some candidates, what next? If your state requires professional licensing, as many states do, ask the massage therapist if he or she is licensed. And ask to *see* the license if you do go for an appointment — just to be safe. (People who are actually licensed are very proud of that fact. They're not hesitant to show you the license, and most of them have it on display on the wall.)

Ask the following questions to the massage therapist you're considering, adding your own questions as well to this list of suggestions:

- ✔ **Have you treated people with fibromyalgia before?** If you get a blank look, that's not a good sign. Move on to someone else who is at least familiar with the term.

  - • If the therapist says he *has* treated people with FMS before, ask him to describe the treatment that he provided.

  - • Also, about how many times did those patients receive massages? (You're looking to find out whether or not this therapist has had any repeat/satisfied customers who have fibromyalgia.)

- ✔ **Do you believe in very vigorous massages only?** If the answer is *yes,* that's the wrong answer for the person with fibromyalgia. Some people gain some benefit by having their bodies pummeled. You won't, and extremely vigorous massage may cause a flare-up of your pain and other symptoms.

✔ **Are you associated with a doctor, chiropractor, or other medical professional in the area?** The massage therapist may have his or her own business, but most have some sort of relationship, even if not a financial one, with a medical professional. If the person says that she works with patients of Dr. Smith, call his office and find out whether they've ever heard of her.

✔ **Is your service covered by health insurance?** Maybe nobody in your area is covered, but this question is still worth asking. Also, you may be pleasantly surprised and find out that your HMO actually will pay for a part of the therapy.

An Electrifying Solution: TENS

Although few clinical studies have backed up the usefulness of TENS, a nerve stimulation therapy, some people report that they gain relief from this treatment. TENS is a noninvasive form of therapy that may work as well for you as it has for others.

Transcutaneous electrical nerve stimulation (TENS) is a machine-based therapy that's designed to deliver low-level electrical impulses to body areas that are in pain or spasm. The goal is to stimulate the nerve tissue to naturally release pain-fighting body chemicals. This treatment is used to help people with fibromyalgia, arthritis, and other medical conditions.

TENS therapy is usually not used in isolation, but, instead, is combined with other pain-relieving techniques or with medications. You may also want to use periodic heat or cold therapy or massage along with your TENS treatments.

The working theory behind TENS

Here's the basic theory to explain why TENS may help people who experience chronic pain: When painful areas of the body are directly stimulated with regular bursts of a very mild electrical current over a short time, these hurting areas of your body are thought to respond to this electrical stimulation by releasing *endorphins*, which are pain-reducing neurochemicals.

These pain-busting chemicals, now thoroughly aroused to action by the external electrical stimulation of the TENS equipment, theoretically rush to the rescue, eventually causing a reduction in both your pain and muscle stiffness. Believers in TENS therapy also think that the stimulated area isn't the only part of the body that responds to the therapy, but that the brain itself also reacts to these periodic electrical impulses, and the end result is diminished pain.

Bedding down in comfort

Some experts say that your choice in bedding is very important. Because you're prone to pain, you may need a special mattress cover like an *egg crate* or one that's made of lambs wool or another material that can "breathe" (you don't want to become sweaty at night and then make the whole problem worse) and also provide you with some extra padding at night. Most people with fibromyalgia have problems with sleeping at night, so a comfortable bed is very important.

What happens during therapy

The physical therapist — or whoever's administering the TENS therapy to you — will apply special small patches with electrodes to your skin directly on the particular areas of your body that are bothering you the most. These patches are connected by wires to a TENS machine. The machine will deliver regular, periodic, and painless pulses of electricity. About 80 to 100 low-level pulses per second are transmitted to TENS patients. Sessions typically last about an hour.

You usually need a calibration in the first treatment, during which the operator will send signals of varying intensity to you to determine when you start to feel anything. People vary in how strong a signal they need; a signal that's weak to other people may be just right or even too strong for you. The goal is for you to feel the electrical impulse but not feel any pain from it.

During the session, you merely lie or sit down and have your painlessly electrifying experience. Don't worry — TENS therapy is nothing like the jolt from a cattle probe or some other painful electrical device, nor is it anywhere near as unsafe. In fact, the electrical impulses emitted by TENS are completely painless. Some people fall asleep during the treatment.

Doing TENS to yourself

Some people purchase or rent portable TENS units, so that they can receive the treatment at home. Your insurance company may be willing to reimburse you for this expense, but you should be sure to check ahead of time before you spend your own money.

The insurance company may have limitations on how much money they'll reimburse you or what types of equipment they'll approve. It would be a shame if you bought your TENS unit from the ABC company, not knowing that your insurance company will only pay for a TENS device from the XYZ company.

The main benefits of having a TENS unit at home are that you won't have to drive to you doctor's or physical therapist's office to receive treatments, and you can manage the treatment yourself in the privacy of your home. You can also arrange to have the treatments during a time that's convenient for you, rather than when you can manage to get an appointment.

The downside of using a TENS unit is that you're probably not trained in this therapy, and will have only the written manual that accompanies the unit to go by. If you experience any problems or discomfort, you won't know if it's normal or abnormal.

Another disadvantage is that TENS units come from many different manufacturers, and deciding which unit is really the best one for you can be difficult. Some units may be hard on the pocketbook, especially if your health insurance company gives you the thumbs down on reimbursing you for the cost of the unit.

Considering Chiropractors

Many people with arthritis or fibromyalgia find small to considerable relief at the hands of a *chiropractor*, a practitioner who "manipulates" the bones and muscle tissues in an effort to relieve pain and stiffness. A chiropractor is not a medical doctor, but he or she is instead a licensed professional who's received specialized training regarding the bones and nervous system.

Chiropractors operate in nearly all states, and many insurance companies provide at least partial medical coverage for their treatments. You may need to obtain approval from your insurance company before the chiropractic treatment may begin, so be sure to check first.

Although most chiropractors are well aware of the need for gentleness when treating FMS patients, if you consult with a chiropractor, you may want to remind him or her that you need to go slow and easy before any treatment begins.

After your diagnosis of FMS has been made by the chiropractor, or she has been informed by you or your doctor that you have fibromyalgia, you should receive a plan of treatment. Massage therapy is often an integral part of the treatment plan of most chiropractors for treating many different medical problems.

Tell the chiropractor about any other medical problems that you may have in addition to your fibromyalgia, such as arthritis, heart disease, osteoporosis, and so forth. This information is important to help tailor your treatment, guiding the chiropractor to go more easily in areas of the body that may be weak.

Be sure to ask the chiropractor the following questions, to which you should add any other questions you may have that are relevant in your particular case:

- ✔ **About how many treatments per week will I need?** The chiropractor should be willing to answer this question without any hesitation, although she may say "about two or three," or "about four or five," or some other approximation.

- ✔ **About how many weeks of treatment will I need?** You may have a more difficult time obtaining an answer to this particular question, but ask it anyway. To be fair, the chiropractor can't really know how many treatments you may need at the beginning of treatment. But he should be able to give you at least a guesstimate. Of course, because fibromyalgia is a chronic illness, treatments will usually be ongoing. More treatments are usually needed at the onset of treatment.

- ✔ **About how many treatments will it take for me to know whether the therapy is working?** This question is another tough one for the chiropractor to answer at the beginning. But ask anyway. You need to know for your own planning. For example, if the chiropractor plans to treat you for six months or longer, but you don't ask and merely assume that treatment will take a month or so, eventually you'll be dissatisfied. It's better to know up front what may be expected down the road.

- ✔ **What can I hope to obtain from this treatment?** If the chiropractor promises you immediate and/or complete relief from your fibromyalgia with his treatments, watch out. Most ethical chiropractors will hope to give you significant relief and improvement in your pain problem, but they won't give you guarantees that you'll be cured.

In addition, make sure that you see the chiropractor's state license. It should be prominently displayed, along with his college degrees and other credentials that are up on the wall. If it's not, ask to see it.

Chapter 12

Considering Alternative Remedies and Treatments

*M*illions of people rely on alternative remedies and treatments to help them with their chronic ailments. So, if you've tried one or even many more forms of alternative medicine to ease your symptoms of fibromyalgia syndrome (FMS), you're definitely not alone!

Whether these alternative therapies come in the form of herbs and supplements, magnets, botox injections, or yet another among the many available alternative solutions today, the fact is that a broad array of nontraditional remedies and treatments have been tried by people with fibromyalgia. Sometimes, people find that these remedies work very well — or at least *seem* to.

On other occasions, people have spent their hard-earned dollars on ridiculous remedies.

They may have known or suspected that these remedies were very silly and would never work, even at the time they purchased them. But they just felt so bad and urgently craved some relief. When you're in major pain and you can't sleep, and a late-night infomercial is advertising Tony Power's Super Fabulous Pain Relief Stuff with Grapefruit Peel Essence, you may think to yourself, "But what if it actually does work? After all, Tony Power obviously feels great!"

Bonnie is one person who's fallen for some of these phony cure-alls. She says that she's tried coffee enemas and many other odd-sounding remedies, and she's also spent thousands of dollars on supplements, which all ended up in the trash. Bonnie says that all the purveyors of alternative remedies told her that they could cure her — but they were all wrong.

But even though you need to be skeptical, don't count out alternative remedies altogether. This chapter helps you separate the alternative therapies that really work — or that may work — from the snake oil that you don't want to spend your money on. When studies are available to back up a form of treatment, I briefly describe them. If a particular alternative remedy has no clinical studies so far, I discuss the treatment from a logical viewpoint.

Thinking Through Alternative Remedies

How can you know if an alternative remedy — whether it's an herb or supplement, acupuncture, or some other therapy that's not considered "mainstream" by your doctors — may help you combat the symptoms of your fibromyalgia? Here are some basic questions to ask yourself about an alternative therapy (whatever it may be) before you try it.

- ✔ **Does the promoter promise that this remedy is an instant cure?** If the answer is *yes,* consider this response to be a red flag. Fibromyalgia has no quick fixes. Maybe one will be found someday, but it's not here yet.

- ✔ **Do you know of anyone who has gained relief from this remedy? If so, how long has he or she tried it?** Often, what seems to work wonderfully for a week or two may prove to be useless in the end. The desire to get better can be so strong that, sometimes, people think that a new remedy will really work, and they actually feel better. This effect usually wears off after awhile, though.

- ✔ **Is the person who's promoting the remedy also selling it?** He or she may be a true proponent, but when they have a financial incentive, think harder before buying the remedy.

- ✔ **Have any recent studies been done on this therapy? If so, were they performed by medical doctors on at least 30 subjects?** Read the abstract (summary) of the study. You can read medical abstracts for free on PubMed, the National Library of Medicine's database at (www.ncbi.nih.gov/entrez/query.fcgi).

- ✔ **Is this therapy safe? What risks are involved?** If the person promoting the therapy says that the therapy has no risks whatsoever, be skeptical. Even drinking too much water can be dangerous, so the therapy most likely has some kind of risk involved with it. You need up-front knowledge of side effects and risks, even if they're very unlikely to occur.

> ✔ **How much is this therapy or treatment going to cost you, and how long will it last?** The price of a remedy that may be "iffy," at best, and how lasting its effects will be should both be key factors in your decision to try a therapy or forego it.

> ✔ **Would this remedy interact with other drugs that your doctor has prescribed? Also, would your doctor disapprove of it?** The best way to find out is to ask your physician. (She may surprise you, and say that the treatment's a good idea.)

Fighting FMS Naturally with Herbs and Supplements

Can taking herbs or supplements make you feel better? When it comes to fibromyalgia, most clinical studies don't show significant results. But experts have made a few positive findings, such as the use of magnesium, taken in combination with another substance or by itself.

Don't forget that you can also combat FMS in more conventional ways. Be sure to read Chapter 9 on over-the-counter remedies that may also help you resolve your fibromyalgia symptoms.

Notifying your doctor about your natural choices

Studies have indicated that many people who decide to try herbal remedies or supplements never discuss that choice with their doctors. They may neglect to mention it for several reasons. Maybe they just forgot to mention it when they saw their physicians. Maybe they assume that all "natural" remedies are safe and, therefore, they don't need to tell the doctor about them. (This assumption is wrong!) Or, maybe they're afraid that the doctor will tell them it's a bad idea, and that they should stop taking it.

Whatever the reason, it's important to overcome it and inform your doctor of the alternative remedies you're taking — or even thinking of taking. Some herbal remedies or supplements can interact with other medications you take, boosting or diminishing their effects.

 Don't get your medical advice from clerks working in health food stores (no matter how knowledgeable they may sound), and don't rely solely on information provided on the label of a supplement or herb that the store is selling. Always check with your physician first before taking any alternative medication to ensure that it's safe for you.

Looking at magnesium

Magnesium is a supplement that everyone needs and that most people obtain in their everyday diet. However, some people are slightly (or very) deficient in magnesium, and this deficiency can lead to serious muscle pain and other symptoms. Magnesium deficiencies have also been associated with migraine headaches and other medical problems.

Magnesium supplements

Some people take magnesium only (as opposed to combinations of magnesium along with other drugs or supplements). Some studies have shown that people who experience migraine headaches and other pain syndromes may have a shortage of magnesium. Even if a person's blood-test levels of magnesium come back as "normal," that person may have a *subclinical,* or slightly below-normal, level of an element. If you're subclinically deficient in magnesium, that shortage could be enough of a problem to contribute to your symptoms of fibromyalgia.

Magnesium supplements are easy to locate — they're available in pharmacies, supermarkets, health food stores, and online. Be sure to check the recommended dosage on the bottle, as well as with your physician. If you take magnesium supplements, keep in mind that magnesium is included in many over-the-counter heartburn remedies, such as Mylanta. If you have a stomachache and take such a drug, you may want to cut back on that day's dose of magnesium.

A couple warnings about magnesium

Avoid overdoing your magnesium intake, whether you're taking a magnesium combination or supplement. Too much magnesium can lead to a shortage of potassium or other minerals that you need. You don't want to unnecessarily create new medical problems while you're trying to resolve your fibromyalgia symptoms. Be sure to take *only* the dose that's recommended on the bottle or the dose that your doctor advises.

You may also find that magnesium causes looser stools or may bring on actual diarrhea. Of course, if you have a problem with chronic constipation that accompanies your fibromyalgia, magnesium may seem like a dream drug to you. It may ease your muscle pain, and also make it possible to have a normal bowel movement. If you're in that situation, what could be better?

Evaluating valerian

Valerian is an herbal remedy that some people take to alleviate their insomnia. (Read more about valerian and its potential impact on overcoming sleep difficulties in Chapter 14.) Valerian may act as a calming drug as well. Some people use valerian to alleviate their stress, as a sort of natural Valium.

TIP

Getting some help that your taxes paid for

The FDA offers many helpful tips on dietary sup-plements, and the basics that you should con-sider before taking these drugs, in their online publication, "Tips for the Savvy Supplement User: Making Informed Decisions and Evaluating Information." Read this publication online at http://vm.cfsan.fda.gov/~dms/ds-savvy.html.

If you decide that you'd like to take valerian for insomnia or stress (or for both), be sure that you follow the directions on the bottle. You should also try this herbal remedy for the first time in the evening or at another time when you won't need to drive a car, operate equipment, or do anything else that requires alertness — just in case valerian causes you to feel very sleepy.

Valerian can be purchased in many pharmacies and supermarkets, as well as in health food stores or online.

Watching out for dangerous remedies

Some natural remedies can be extremely dangerous, particularly some drugs that purport to help you lose weight but that are primarily comprised of highly stimulating drugs (such as *ephedra* or *ma huang*). The effects of such drugs are similar to the action of an excessive level of the hormone adrena-line. These drugs may act like a nonprescription amphetamine drug, speeding up your metabolism to dangerous, or even fatal, levels. The *Food and Drug Administration* (FDA) has issued consumer warnings against using these drugs or any drugs that contain ephedra or ma huang.

Some supplements can cause adverse effects and should be avoided by some patients altogether, and by other people in certain situations. For example, *gingko biloba* thins the blood, and people who also take blood thinners, such as Coumadin (generic name: warfarin), should not take this substance. Gingko biloba should *never* be taken by anyone before surgery or a medical procedure.

If you note any negative effect that may have been caused by a supplement, call MedWatch, a toll-free number offered by the FDA. The phone number is 800-FDA-1088. Or you can contact the FDA online at: www.fda.gov/mcdwatch/how.htm

Pinning Down a Solution: Acupuncture

Some people with fibromyalgia announce feeling considerable relief after undergoing *acupuncture*, the careful insertion of special pins at specific points of the body by a trained practitioner. Others, however, have said that acupuncture had no effect on them, and some have reported that the experience made them feel worse.

Acupuncture therapy may or may not be covered by your health insurance, and you should check with them ahead of time to find out. If your health insurance company *does* cover acupuncture treatments, keep in mind that your acupuncture sessions are far more likely to be covered when the person performing the acupuncture is a medical doctor, osteopathic physician, or a nurse practitioner.

Deciding whether acupuncture can make a difference

So far, clinical studies on acupuncture have provided mixed results on whether it's an effective therapy in treating fibromyalgia and other medical problems. Some studies have shown that acupuncture doesn't work any better than taking a *placebo* (a sugar pill with no medicine in it). In other words, acupuncture may help your fibromyalgia about as much as one piece of candy would.

Other studies, however, indicate that people *have* found significant relief from acupuncture.

For example, research that was presented in 2001 at the annual meeting of the American College of Rheumatology revealed positive results from acupuncture. The effect of acupuncture was tested on 40 women diagnosed with fibromyalgia.

Twenty of the women received 30-minute acupuncture sessions once a week. Another 20 women received sham acupuncture, in which they were punctured in areas that the researchers believed would have no effect on pain. The patients who received the real acupuncture reported that they experienced significant decreases in their pain, while the woman receiving sham acupuncture didn't have significant pain reductions. These effects lasted for about four months after the treatment ended, after which time the improvement began to decline.

As of this writing, the National Institutes of Health (NIH) in the United States is overseeing clinical studies at several locations to determine whether acupuncture may prove to be a beneficial therapy in treating patients who have fibromyalgia.

No needling me!

Acupressure is a form of therapy that uses direct pressure, but it doesn't penetrate the skin like the pins used in acupuncture do. Instead, noninvasive (and nonpin) firm pressure is applied to the particular areas of your body that hurt. You can perform acupressure on yourself by pressing on your sore areas (assuming that you can reach those painful areas). For areas that you can't easily reach, such as your middle or lower back, some people suggest that your acupressurize yourself by lying on top of a tennis ball and moving around on it.

Understanding acupuncture

The Chinese have explanations about acupuncture that are fairly complicated and may make little sense to the Western mind. So I'll stick to one possible explanation of acupuncture that may be feasible and more understandable to the average American. That explanation is that if and when acupuncture works, the pins that are inserted may stimulate the production of *endorphins*, or pain-fighting neurochemicals.

Because your pain actually preceded the acupuncture treatment, why weren't those endorphins already working beforehand? Didn't your body know that it was hurting and should have marshaled your endorphins to get to work? No one knows why pain sometimes seems to get stuck in the "on" mode.

Acupuncture may give your system that extra little jolt that's enough to stimulate the endorphins to rush to the hurting area. When endorphins go up, pain goes down. Acupuncture is only a temporary fix at best. But then, few remedies that are associated with fibromyalgia are long-term solutions.

Finding an acupuncturist

You can ask your physician or your friends to recommend an acupuncturist, but, sometimes, they may disapprove of your plan. Even if they feel neutral or okay about it, they may not know of an acupuncture practitioner. Another alternative is to check the yellow pages of the phone book under "acupuncture" and look for ads there. Are any of the practitioners medical doctors? Start with them.

If you're also considering an acupuncturist who's not a medical doctor or an osteopathic physician, make sure that any individual you're considering is licensed by the state. Check with the state department of professional regulation, usually based in the state capital. Then, be sure that you at least first talk to that person on the phone before going for an appointment. Although many non-medical acupuncture practitioners are honest people who know what they're doing, some of them may regard acupuncture as an easy way to make a few bucks.

You should avoid such people! One obvious reason why you should stay away from people trying to get rich quick is that they may also be very careless. In order to save money, they may reuse the acupuncture needles.

Reusing needles is an absolute no-no in acupuncture therapy, and it places you at risk for contracting hepatitis or the HIV virus that leads to AIDS, as well as too many other infectious diseases to mention. The probability that someone would take this risk seems low, but patients need to consider worst-case scenarios and protect themselves as much as possible.

I'm not saying that the *only* good acupuncturist is a person with a medical degree. I'm just saying that you should put on your best skeptical thinking cap and your good listening ears, and you should ask plenty of questions before signing up for acupuncture treatments with someone who isn't a doctor. (Actually, you should also ask plenty of questions even if the acupuncture practitioner *is* a medical doctor.)

Some questions to consider asking an acupuncturist are:

- ✔ How long have you been performing acupuncture? (More than a year would be desirable.)

- ✔ Are you affiliated with a medical doctor or a chiropractor? ("Yes" is better than "no" because it means that someone is at least periodically checking on them. You should also verify with the doctor or chiropractor that he or she does in fact have a business relationship with the acupuncturist. Some people make statements because they don't believe that others will check up on them. Check up.)

- ✔ How many sessions will it take for me to feel better, if it works for me? (If the acupuncturist says daily for weeks, that's too many. At most, several times a week at the start of therapy should be sufficient.)

- ✔ Do you guarantee that this procedure will make me feel better? (If the person says "yes," leave. No competent person will issue blanket guarantees.)

To obtain a listing of medical doctors and osteopathic physicians in your area who perform acupuncture on patients, contact the *American Academy of Medical Acupuncture* at their toll-free number (800-521-2262) or search their Web site (www.medicalacupuncture.org).

Beating FMS with Botox Injections

One of the newer and somewhat controversial remedies that doctors sometimes use to treat people with fibromyalgia is the injection of botox. *Botox* is a form of the botulinum toxin, which is a kind of a poison that's created by a specific bacterium, *Clostridium botulinum.* At least seven or eight different forms of botox are used to treat a wide array of medical problems.

The doses of botox that are used are considered to be small enough to avoid harming the patient, but, at the same time, they're also large enough to provide noticeable results with a problem of the nervous system or of the musculoskeletal system.

Physicians use botox to treat many different types of medical problems, such as tremors, tics, stroke, cerebral palsy, multiple sclerosis, chronic low back or neck pain, chronic headaches, and a wide variety of other medical conditions. Some plastic surgeons also use botox to cosmetically (and temporarily) rid people of their facial wrinkles.

Physicians who are open to using acupuncture, as well as other alternative treatments, may also be more open to using botox therapy. Doctors who are pain-management experts and neurologists are probably more likely to consider using botox therapy, although there's no uniformity on which particular specialty of doctors use botox on their patients and which don't.

Doctors who treat patients with botox injections should have previous experience with using this therapy, particularly when using botox with their patients who have fibromyalgia and who are very pain sensitive. Don't let someone practice on you! In addition, the physician should also be someone whom you feel that you can fully trust with using this new form of therapy on you.

In the hands of an inexperienced and incompetent practitioner who may inject too high a dose or make other medical errors, botox treatments can theoretically cause a temporary paralysis or even result in more severe harm to some patients. This risk is yet another reason to make sure that you receive your botox treatments only from a doctor knowledgeable and experienced in the procedure.

A healthful bacteria

Most people spend a lot of time trying to *avoid* bacteria, carefully washing their hands with antibacterial soap, taking daily baths or showers, and trying to keep their bodies and their clothes as clean as they can. For the most part, bacteria are seen as being bad and something to avoid. Botox is created by bacteria, and consequently, the idea of injecting it into your system may make you feel a little squeamish. It may almost sound like injecting dirt.

Yet, when you really think about it, not all bacteria are bad. For one simple example, bacteria in your stomach enable you to digest your food more easily by helping to break it down. When you take antibiotics to combat an infection that you have (such as a strep throat or a urinary tract infection), those bacteria may be killed, or at least weakened, and thus, you get diarrhea and can't digest your food as well.

You may also develop a yeast infection while you're taking antibiotics because the bacteria that have been killed by the antibiotic were also the ones that had previously kept the yeast at bay. They're gone, so the yeast can proliferate. So, it's not exactly true that the only good bacteria are dead bacteria.

Botox and FMS

Botox treatments for people with fibromyalgia are a relatively new form of therapy. But botox use may explode in the next few years, particularly if both clinical research and patients' word of mouth indicate that botox can provide the pain relief that patients so desperately want and need. In fact, it could really take off if the prices were to come down.

Joseph Kandel, MD, a neurologist and the medical director of Neuroscience and Spine Associates in Naples, Florida, has treated numerous patients with fibromyalgia with botox treatments. Dr. Kandel says that botox injections can be quite successful in treating the muscle changes, muscle spasms, and the general spasticity that many patients with fibromyalgia experience.

Dr. Kandel says that the relief that's provided by a botox injection may last anywhere from a few weeks to a few months, depending on the individual patient. During that temporary period, the patient (hopefully) will experience at least a partial reprieve from their severe pain, and this will allow him or her to exercise and to increase range of motion and muscle function. These actions can then help patients to prevent, or at least delay, a further flare-up in problem areas.

Using botox in pain management is a relatively new application. The use of botox in fibromyalgia has not been sufficiently studied in clinical tests to determine whether it's a useful therapy. Doctors who do favor botox say that it works for a majority, but not all, of their patients. So don't expect any guarantees if you sign up for botox injections. (For that matter, don't expect guarantees with any other medical procedures that you receive, either.)

As of this writing, the FDA hasn't approved botox injections to treat chronic pain from fibromyalgia or any other chronic pain condition. This approval may come in the near future, but it's not here yet. Despite this fact, doctors may still legally administer the injections.

Nerving yourself for neurofeedback

Neurofeedback is a treatment option that, theoretically, enables its users to master their own brain wave patterns. The idea is that after brain wave patterns are identified, subjects can then obtain mastery over their fibromyalgia symptoms. However, some other forms of neurofeedback don't require any particular mastery over brain wave patterns. Instead, everything is supposedly done by your brain at the unconscious level, and no conscious effort is required.

Neurofeedback is different from biofeedback, which is described in Chapter 13. With biofeedback, users concentrate on lowering their blood pressure, pulse, and body temperature to achieve a relaxed state. In contrast, with neurofeedback, users try to change actual brain waves.

It sounds very mysterious — almost occult-like in nature. But the physicians and other experts who support neurofeedback as a treatment for fibromyalgia and other chronic pain problems say that it can be extremely effective, although sufficient clinical research has yet to be performed to fully back up the effectiveness of neurofeedback.

Researchers (such as Jeff Hargrove, PhD, an assistant professor of engineering at Kettering University in Flint, Michigan, and an adjunct assistant professor of medicine with the Department of Medicine at Michigan State University) are currently in the process of overseeing investigative studies on using neurofeedback devices.

Hargrove says that many experts believe that the root of the dysfunction in fibromyalgia lies in the brain and in electrical abnormalities that are found there. As a result, if the electrical stimulation of parts of the brain can in some way counteract these abnormalities, as is hoped with neurofeedback (also known as EEG stimulation), this encounter may lead to symptomatic improvements.

How much botox costs and whether insurance pays

If you're currently considering botox therapy, keep in mind that this form of therapy is generally not the low-cost or the bargain-basement option, and if you have a shortage of dollars, you may not even be able to afford it. In general, botox is more like the upscale, probably-not-covered-by-your-health-insurance form of treatment — although this situation may be changing soon because some insurance companies have started to provide payments for botox treatment. If and when the FDA approves botox as a therapy for chronic pain, more health insurance providers will likely cover such treatments.

Most patients need to receive at least two vials of botox to gain a sufficient amount of the substance to obtain relief from their chronic pain, and one vial costs about $500. As a result, in considering all the costs involved, a botox procedure can cost at least $1,000 and can go much higher than that.

However, proponents say that when botox injections work to resolve symptoms, patients won't need lots of doctor visits, and they can also avoid taking many doses of pain medications and, thus, avoid enduring their side effects. Looking at it from that point of view, botox injections may be cost-effective treatments for some fibromyalgia patients.

As for whether health insurance will pay for botox to treat your fibromyalgia, the answer is usually "no," at least for now. Whether health insurance company officials admit it or not, they usually don't like things that fall under the "expensive" category, and they usually aren't that crazy about "new" either. Even worse, they hate "expensive" and "new" when they go together.

In a few years, botox treatments may be readily covered by your health insurance carrier, who will cover it without batting an eyelash, but don't assume that that time is right now. On the other hand, don't assume that it's not. Always check first by simply calling and asking your insurance company if botox treatments are covered.

Taking On T'ai Chi

The gentle art of the basic Chinese exercise movements of T'ai Chi are usually not overly difficult to master, and generally these movements can also be a very good form of exercise for people who have fibromyalgia or other chronic pain problems. The basic exercises are meant to resemble natural animal movements, such as movements that may be made by a crane, a tiger, a snake, or other animals. For example, one simple T'ai Chi movement involves standing on one leg as a crane would.

T'ai Chi helps patients with FMS in two basic ways: The exercises are relatively easy to perform for people with muscle problems who find it difficult to perform more arduous exercises. Also, the exercises can help with relaxation, in a meditative sort of way.

T'ai Chi movements are also considered low-impact exercises, and consequently, they generally involve very little risk for the person who's practicing them. In fact, T'ai Chi exercises are even recommended for elderly and sick people who are living in nursing homes — so how hard can they be for the rest of us? You may also find that regular practicing of the basic T'ai Chi exercises can help to considerably ease the pain and fatigue of your fibromyalgia.

How do you master T'ai Chi? You can often take classes on T'ai Chi movements at a community center or at your fitness club; check your local newspapers for mentions of classes. Or you may also want to supplement your knowledge with *T'ai Chi For Dummies*, by Therese Iknoian and Manny Fuentes (published by Wiley), a helpful book that can show you all the ropes.

Repelling Magnet Therapy

Some people believe that using magnetized necklaces, bracelets, earrings, or even magnetic bed mattresses — as well as magnets in many other forms — can somehow help to decrease their pain. Sadly, a review of the existing evidence on magnet therapy indicates that magnets really *don't* provide any significant pain relief for people with fibromyalgia or other diseases with chronic pain. It would be nice if they did, but the truth is, they simply don't work.

Be a skeptical reader when you come across ads or even articles about non-traditional therapies, particularly when you read about claims for "magnet therapy." Despite the dramatic ad copy, complete with many testimonials, and despite the rhetoric that sounds really scientific (although it's usually written in such a way that few people could make any sense out of it), keep in mind that magnet therapy is a no-sale when it comes to pain relief for fibromyalgia.

If you do use magnets to help your pain, fatigue, and other symptoms of fibromyalgia and find that you really are feeling better, you're most likely experiencing the *placebo effect*. In other words, you intensely hoped and believed that the therapy would work for you, and so, for a short time, your fervent desire for symptomatic relief seemed to make magnet therapy improve your condition.

After awhile, however, your mind and your pain will both overcome your wishful thinking, and you'll be right back to where you started: hurting again. (And minus the bucks that you paid out for all the magnetized paraphernalia.)

Will magnet therapy hurt you in any way at all? Probably not. No evidence suggests that using magnets will be harmful to you — *unless* you decide that you'll completely substitute magnet therapy for your medication or for other treatments that can provide you with real pain improvement.

Honing in on homeopathy

In 2001, the National Institutes of Health (NIH) awarded a grant to study the effectiveness of *homeopathy,* a form of alternative/complementary medicine that's based on the belief that extremely small doses of herbs can improve health. As part of the study, homeopathy will be practiced on patients with fibromyalgia. The Society for the Establishment of Research in Classical Homeopathy (SERCH) in Phoenix, Arizona, will conduct a two-year study, which will help determine what type of individuals respond best to homeopathy. Another purpose of the study is to determine if homeopathy should be studied on a larger scale in the future.

Study subjects will be treated with homeopathy for six months, and their responses will be evaluated to see if homeopathy can really help patients with fibromyalgia.

Smelling Your Way to Health with Aromatherapy

Perhaps inhaling the scent of lovely flowers or other pleasant smells can help improve your overall condition, or at least temporarily elevate your mood state. Proponents of *aromatherapy*, or using odors to improve general health, are quite convinced that this possibility is true.

As a physician and a scientist, I can't recommend aromatherapy as a stand-alone therapeutic choice for fibromyalgia unless and until clinical studies are performed that prove that patients show actual benefit from its use. At the present, no clinically acceptable studies have been done that support (or refute) the use of aromatherapy as a viable treatment for the various symptoms of fibromyalgia.

At the same time, aromatherapy is very unlikely to be harmful to you (except, perhaps, to your pocketbook, depending on what products you buy and how much of them), and you may really enjoy experimenting with the different types of scents that are offered in aromatherapy.

If you're interested, you can purchase aromatherapy products in many different places. Even local pharmacies and supermarkets now offer many different types of fragrances that are available in the form of candles, incense, beads, and many other options.

You may want to consult with an aromatherapy expert in your area. Ask your local health food store for the names of people to contact in your area who are knowledgeable about aromatherapy choices. Do keep in mind that the practice of aromatherapy is generally an area that is not state licensed or regulated. Don't look for any serious science with aromatherapy, as of this writing.

If you'd like to find out more about aromatherapy, for a comprehensive overview, read *Aromatherapy For Dummies,* by Kathi Keville (Wiley).

Part IV
Lifestyle Changes: What You Can Do on Your Own

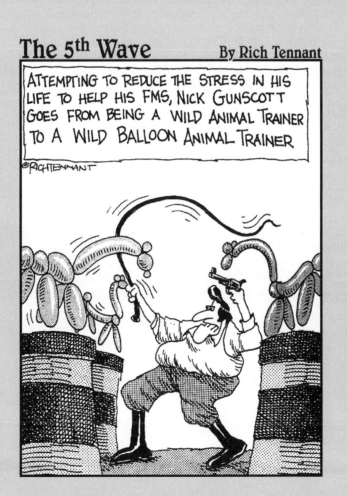

In this part . . .

A lot of people want to decrease their pain and the other symptoms related to fybromyalgia even further than they can by simply taking the medication their doctors prescribe. They want to take action. I agree! I recommend plenty of good lifestyle changes for patients with fibromyalgia, and I include them all in Part IV. For example, most people with fibromyalgia are unbelievably stressed out, even more so than the average person without fibromyalgia. Reduce the stress, and you ease your symptoms, which is why I devote Chapter 13 to "depressurizing" yourself.

Increasing your amount of quality sleep time is another good lifestyle change. Many people with fibromyalgia are insomniacs or have other sleep problems, which worsens their symptoms. I address these issues in Chapter 14. I also cover the importance of exercising (it can be fun if it's an activity you like — and yes, you can find a physical activity that you like), paying attention to weight issues, and avoiding foods that can trigger symptoms. You get all this in one chapter: Chapter 15. Then I discuss your emotions, which are often pretty ragged from the pain, fatigue, and other symptoms. So I tell you what to do about those emotional valleys in Chapter 16.

Chapter 13

Depressurizing Yourself: Controlling the Stress-Eyed Monster

Did you ever think that you'd need help relaxing? Can't you simply just "let go" and relax yourself at will — take a vacation, go see a movie, do something else that you enjoy to make the stress evaporate like dew before the morning sun? It'd be wonderful if unwinding from life's stresses were that easy. But often, it's not.

Most people really don't know how to relax. They may *think* that they know how, but very often, the means that they choose to relax themselves can be useless or even harmful.

If you think that I'm exaggerating, let me give you a few common examples of some of the major means that people use to "relax": alcohol, chocolate cake (or chocolate anything), going to visit the in-laws. (Just kidding about that last one, which is a stress creator for many people!)

In this chapter, I explain several effective ways that you can relax by using various stress-busting techniques. When you use these techniques to de-stress, you also help to diminish your fibromyalgia syndrome (FMS) symptoms — because stress and fibromyalgia *are* related.

The stress-pain connection in FMS

Studies indicate that people with fibromyalgia are much more prone to suffering from stress than other people are, and that this increased vulnerability to stress worsens their fibromyalgia-related pain. One study, reported in a 2001 issue of the *Annals of Behavioral Medicine*, asked 101 women, including women with fibromyalgia and women with severe knee pain from osteoarthritis, about their stress. The researchers found that the women with FMS reported much greater levels of stress than the women with severe osteoarthritis.

In a related study, researchers purposely *caused* the women with fibromyalgia and those with osteoarthritis only to experience stress by having them discuss stressful events. The researchers found that the women with FMS experienced increased pain with stress, but the women who had osteoarthritis were not similarly affected. Stress doesn't cause pain, but for women with fibromyalgia, it clearly can make it much worse.

Knowing When You're Too Stressed

Maybe you don't think that you're really all that stressed out, or at least no more than most of the other people that you know at work or at home. But, sometimes, when people feel the same bad way for a long time, they don't even realize that they can feel better — sometimes, much better. This skewed perspective is certainly true for overly stressed people. You may have forgotten what feeling plain-old normal is like. How do you know?

Reading through the list that follows can help you determine just how stressed you are. This list isn't really a test, where you answer *true* or *false,* and then I tell you exactly what to do based on your answers. But it should get you thinking about how much stress you really have in your life.

- **I frequently berate the driving of other people when I drive. They all drive like total morons.** If you spend most of your driving time ridiculing the driving of others, and screaming and yelling at these people who can't hear you, you're probably stressed out. Sure, some of the drivers are probably annoying or even incompetent. But most of them are, at least, average. Maybe the problem is your underlying stress, which you're taking out on others who can't argue back.

- **Nearly every morning when I wake up, I'm worried about whether I'll be able to get everything done.** If your first thought upon waking up in the morning is to worry about getting all your many tasks done, you're not hitting the day running. You're hitting the day crashing and burning. Everyone worries sometimes. But you need to take a moment to chill out, including in the a.m.

✔ **I feel like everyone is demanding too much of me, and I'm being torn apart.** You may feel like your partner wants things from you, your family members are demanding other things, and your boss wants something else. You feel like the rope in a game of emotional tug-of-war. That's stress.

✔ **If my boss asks me to do just one more thing, I think I'll explode.** You may think that you have too do much to do as it is, but while you're trying to do what you're supposed to do, your boss keeps loading you down with even more work. It's maddening! If you feel terribly over-loaded and your boss is unsympathetic, take a deep breath and work on relaxation. Therapy may also help you deal with your anger, even when it's well-placed anger.

✔ **My family members care about my problems and try to help me as much as they can.** That's good! A caring family can go a long way to reduce stress. If you *don't* think that your family is caring and support-ive, however, you may have a problem with stress. This is true whether you're right about your uncaring family or wrong, and they really *do* care. (Perception can cloud out reality.) However, for some people, a caring and helpful family can be a stress inducer — if you're worried that your child is doing too much for you or if you're an overachiever and you can't stand it that others are doing things for you that you think you should be doing yourself.

✔ **As soon as I get home, I make a beeline for the liquor cabinet or a six-pack in the fridge.** If you feel so overwhelmed by work and/or family problems that you head for some (alcoholic) liquid refreshment at the slightest provocation, you need to be concerned about your stress levels. Many people think that alcohol is the answer for stress relief, but if you're emotionally or physically dependent on it, it isn't. Work on de-stressing your life, using various healthy techniques, instead. And get some help for the alcohol dependency.

✔ **On a scale of 1 to 10, with 10 being best, my life is a –5.** This one is a little silly, asking if your life could be rated in the negative numbers on a scale of 1 to 10. However, if you nodded your head when you read this, you're experiencing entirely too much stress in your life.

✔ **I can't remember when I've been to a nonbusiness dinner or done anything that's fun.** Doing things just for fun is a normal part of life. If you can't remember the last night you had a nonbusiness dinner, went to the movie, or just plain did something fun, then face it: You're sad-dling yourself with too much stress. Don't have any time for fun? You need to *make* and *take* the time. Doing so pays off in reduced symptoms of stress and fibromyalgia.

✔ **I've been averaging about eight hours of sleep a night.** That's great! Sleep problems are a major factor for many people with fibromyalgia. However, if you get less than eight hours of sleep a night, you need to work on that problem. A good night's sleep can help you de-stress and reduce your symptoms. (Read Chapter 14 for more information on sleep and fibromyalgia.)

✔ **Sometimes, I worry that the boss will fire me. Sometimes, I worry that he won't, and I'll have to do this job for the rest of my life.** If you constantly worry about getting fired, you're under some stress. You may also be suffering from problems with anxiety and depression as well. If you sometimes wish that your boss *would* fire you (because you have such an awful job), there's probably nothing wrong with you. And if you really hate your job this much, isn't it time to just look for another one? Feeling trapped in a job can increase your stress levels tremendously.

Chilling Out with Relaxation Therapy

Relaxation therapy is a strategy that uses steps to achieve a calming of both the body and the mind. In general, the person consciously concentrates on relaxing one part of the body, or one set of muscles, at a time until the entire body is in a state of relaxation. The great thing about relaxation therapy is that you can practice it on your own at home as often as you want.

Here's how it works: Close the blinds or pull down the shades (if darkness helps you relax, as it does for many people). Then lie down and begin the therapy.

You can really start by relaxing any part of your body, as long as you concentrate, focus, and work to *completely* relax that part of your body. For example, you may choose to start at your feet.

In this case, you start by imagining your feet becoming increasingly relaxed, loose, and tension-free. You breathe deeply and tell yourself, in your mind, that your feet are becoming heavy and too hard to hold up. Then you imagine this relaxed feeling slowly moving its way up your body to the knees and then to the upper leg. Keep telling yourself that each part of the body is heavy and needs (and *wants*) to rest.

Take your time. You can't rush through relaxation therapy. Don't move on to another part of your body until the part that you're concentrating on feels completely relaxed.

The relaxation mode continues up through the trunk of your body and out into your arms. You may choose to end with your head and your very, very tired eyes that just want to close. Or, you may want to close your eyes at the very beginning of your relaxation session. Either way can work.

If relaxation therapy can help with heartburn, it can help with FMS

In 1994, researchers reported on the results of training people who suffer from severe chronic heartburn in relaxation therapy in *Gastroenterology*, a journal for physicians specializing in digestive diseases. Chronic heartburn? What's that got to do with fibromyalgia? Just bear with me for a moment.

The researchers had inserted special instruments in the stomachs of the subjects, so that they could actually measure each person's stomach acidity when the experiment began, and then again when it ended. Then they trained subjects in one group to perform relaxation therapy, while the other group watched a movie. Both groups were given the same heartburn-inducing meals. (Pepperoni pizza with extra cheese and cola to drink.)

So what happened? The relaxation therapy group experienced a significant reduction in the level of acidity in their stomachs, and they also felt much better. The other group, which didn't receive the relaxation training, suffered from significantly higher levels of stomach acidity, and they also experienced heartburn.

The researchers hypothesized that maybe the deep breathing that was part of the relaxation therapy helped people with heartburn feel better. Or maybe the relaxation itself somehow reduced the production of acid.

The point, and the relationship to fibromyalgia is this one: Relaxation therapy had a pronounced effect in this study, such that people somehow unknowingly reduced their stomach acid by practicing relaxation therapy, So, isn't it also possible that relaxation therapy may help reduce some of *your* troubling symptoms of fibromyalgia, such as pain, morning stiffness, and sleep problems? Certainly, relaxation therapy seems to be well worth a try.

You may notice that relaxation therapy uses some of the basic techniques that are also used in hypnotherapy; however, with relaxation therapy, relaxation is the goal. With hypnotherapy, relaxation is merely the path to get to the goal, which is to adopt suggestions that are given to you while you're under hypnosis.

Some people accompany their relaxation "self-talk" with thinking about a pleasant place where they'd feel relaxed. Some people imagine resting in a quiet forest; others may equate relaxation with thinking about the crashing of the ocean's waves or another scene. You're bounded only by your own imagination.

If you think that relaxation therapy sounds like nonsense, try making a deal with yourself. You want to find a way to feel more relaxed, with less fatigue, stiffness, and pain, right? So why not give relaxation therapy at least one or two tries? What have you got to lose? If it doesn't work, you haven't done yourself any harm or even wasted any money. And if it does work, you've gained a new strategy to cope with your stress and, perhaps, lessen your FMS pain.

You can purchase a relaxation audiotape to help you discover everything you'd ever need to know about relaxation therapy. Some stores even let you listen to relaxation audiotapes before you decide to buy one. Listen for a voice you find appealing and soothing. Avoid tapes that offer *subliminal messages*, or messages heard only unconsciously. They may work, but the goal is to figure out how to achieve relaxation on your own, and when you don't have the tape available.

Stress-busting with Biofeedback Therapy

When most people become upset or angry, their bodies react with raised blood pressure and pulse and with changes in skin temperature as well. They may remain angry or upset for a long time, which worsens their fibromyalgia symptoms of pain, fatigue, sleep difficulties, and so on.

You can work on what's bothering you with "talk therapy," by discussing it with a therapist. Or, another option is to master the art of controlling and changing your own body responses. It's hard to stay upset when your blood pressure and pulse drop, your breathing steadies, and your body temperature stabilizes.

Can you really control your body changes, such as lowering your blood pressure, dropping your skin temperature, and making other physical changes? Supporters of *biofeedback* (a therapy that works to enable the user to change his or her body responses through concentration and observation of physical changes on a computer screen) think that *yes,* you can. And they also believe that biofeedback training can enable you to become more focused and more relaxed.

What happens

Different biofeedback practitioners use different methods, but in general, the patient sits in a chair and is connected to a series of monitors. One monitor takes the skin temperature of the hand or arm. Another monitor, often placed on a finger, takes the pulse. Other monitors may also be used to take various body measurements, such as your blood pressure.

The individual views a representation (often a line graph) of temperature or pulse on a monitor, and is told to relax. As the person relaxes, he can see the measures dropping down. As he relaxes further, the line also drops as well. If the person gets agitated, the line starts to climb up.

When it works, biofeedback enables a person to learn to decrease these various measures of stress. By doing so, that person can achieve a better state of relaxation, which he can duplicate when he's not hooked up to monitors and machines.

That's the theory, anyway. It doesn't always work, particularly with "Type A" achievers who are more likely to see the graph take a downturn and automatically become excited, causing stress levels to rise. For some people, equating relaxation with success is very difficult.

Some studies of the results of biofeedback have indicated that patients with fibromyalgia have decreased their pain, fatigue, and morning stiffness and also improved their sleep.

Perhaps one reason why biofeedback may work for people with fibromyalgia is that studies of people with FMS have indicated that they have temperature differences as well as differences in the blood flow, compared to people who don't have fibromyalgia. If the problem is body responses, and you can discover how to change your physical responses, you may also be able to master your fibromyalgia symptoms. This ability to control your physical responses doesn't mean that you can cure yourself of all pain and fatigue forever. But if biofeedback works for you, it may give you an edge, and a way to improve how you feel.

Weighing the pros and cons of biofeedback therapy

As you may expect, biofeedback therapy has both benefits and liabilities. Let me start with the "bad news." First, your health insurance company may not provide coverage, so the sessions can be pricey. Second, identifying a trained professional who has the equipment and who is competent to provide the therapy may be difficult. Third, the therapy also takes time. Biofeedback improvements may not occur in the first few sessions, and it may take longer than you'd like before you see any results — not a good thing if you're paying out of pocket for these treatments.

A reminder: Rest!

Taking time out for some rest and relaxation is not a bad thing, although one might think that it is in our hyperactive society where the cultural concentration is centered on working harder and faster. Your body and your mind need diversions. At least once every few days, do something fun or take some time to do nothing at all. Doing nothing involves activities like listening to gentle music, or watching birds outside your window, or taking a bubble bath. Plan for this kind of down time in your schedule because it's good for your body and for your soul.

Don't watch television to relax, and if you do watch TV, stop watching it at least 30 minutes before you want to go to bed. Watching TV (or playing on your computer) causes the electrical activity of the brain to increase, and makes relaxation and sleep more difficult to achieve.

The major pro is that if biofeedback therapy works, you'll feel better. Experts also believe that you can generalize the results of biofeedback to your daily life. That is, after you've mastered the technique, you no longer need to be hooked up to a machine that measures your blood pressure, pulse, and so forth. Instead, when you feel yourself starting to stress out, you can (at least, theoretically) call upon the capabilities that you've gained through the biofeedback training. In one study, patients were still successful at using what they'd learned even six months after biofeedback therapy had completely ended. They hadn't forgotten the techniques, even though they were no longer receiving the treatments.

Finding biofeedback providers

In general, psychologists and therapists are the primary people who provide biofeedback therapy to the stressed-out individuals who need it. They have the equipment, and they have the training to know how to use it correctly and to help you mobilize your abilities. You can ask your physician and others you know if they can recommend anyone with training in biofeedback therapy. If you live near a university or major hospital, you can call the public relations staff to find out if they know of any biofeedback practitioners.

Mesmerizing the Pain: Hypnotherapy

Look deeply into my eyes! You're getting sleepy, very sleepy. Most people think of hypnotherapy in terms of a rather scary-looking person who somehow makes them fall into his or her "power" and induces them to lose weight or rid themselves of other bad habits. Or they may perceive hypnosis as something fake and useless — a carnival trick — and nothing more.

Although, sadly, plenty of charlatans *are* out there in the business, claiming to offer hypnosis services but selling only lies, many other people in the business actually do provide a genuine service. Hypnosis (done correctly) really can help some people gain better control over their lives, helping them to become more calm (and not zombified!), lose weight, stop smoking, or alter their other bad habits.

Hypnosis has other possible applications as well, and one practical possibility (if it works) is to assist you with getting to sleep or gaining some control over your pain. Hypnosis has been used successfully to calm people who need painful medical or dental procedures, and even to help cancer patients who need to control their pain. Hypnosis can be very helpful with pain management for many conditions, including fibromyalgia.

In fact, hypnotherapy has been shown to work for some patients with fibromyalgia. For example, in a study of patients with fibromyalgia treated with hypnotherapy or physical therapy (reported in a 1991 issue of the *Journal of Rheumatology*), researchers found that the patients who received 12 weeks of hypnotherapy reported better sleep, less fatigue, and less pain than the subjects who'd received physical therapy. The benefits were sustained for six months after the end of the hypnotherapy.

Considering what hypnosis is and isn't

Hypnosis is an altered state of consciousness. It isn't a state of sleep, but it isn't exactly a state of being awake, either. Contrary to any myths that you may have heard about hypnosis, it's not some magic trick that's performed on you to make you do stupid things that you aren't aware of. A hypnotist can't compel you to have sex with him or murder his wife or do anything that you'd consider objectionable or dangerous. A hypnotist may, however, be able to help you to marshal your inner resources to figure out how to relax as well as lose weight, quit smoking, and conquer other bad habits.

Knowing exactly what goes on during hypnotherapy

Hypnosis creates a passive, relaxed state, and during that state, the person is receptive to suggestions that can benefit their needs or goals. During a hypnotherapy session, the hypnotist has the patient sit back or lie down. Often, the individual closes her eyes. The hypnotist uses some relaxation therapy techniques, such as telling the person that her feet are very tired, then her knees, and so on. The hypnotist may tell the person that on the count of ten, she will be extremely relaxed.

The hypnotist may then tell the person that she can't open her eyes, and then tell the person to try to open her eyes, even though she can't. If the person struggles to open her eyes, but fails, she's in a hypnotic trance. If her eyes fly open, she isn't, and more effort needs to be done to achieve a light trance.

In most cases, the hypnotist tailors the session to the problem to be addressed. For example, if stress reduction is the goal, the hypnotist may tell the person to imagine a place where she felt really calm, happy, and serene. The hypnotist may tell her to think about how she felt, what the scene appeared like, what sounds she heard, and so forth. The person may be told that she's in this place, and she's very happy. She may be told that when she's feeling very stressed out, she should think about this place, and she'll begin to feel calmer and more relaxed.

Locating a hypnotherapist

You may want to ask your physician if she can recommend a hypnotist — keeping in mind that many doctors consider hypnosis a dubious procedure, at best. You can also locate therapists who've been trained and certified in hypnotherapy through your state or local psychological and psychiatric associations. So, you don't have to let your doctor's negative opinion of hypnosis prevent you from finding a qualified hypnotherapist.

Mastering self-hypnosis

Maybe you'd prefer to take charge and figure out how to perform hypnosis on yourself. But how on earth can you first put yourself "under" and then, at the same time, give yourself hypnotic suggestions? It may sound impossible, but experts say that self-hypnosis is doable.

One possibility is to use a tape recording of your voice with the suggestions that want to reinforce in your mind. Another possibility is to sort of "pre-program" your mind with the ideas and concepts that you want to concentrate upon, such as imaging your body as healthy, strong, and with little or no pain. Use your relaxation therapy techniques to achieve a state of relaxation, and then introduce the positive goals that you want to achieve.

For further information on self-hypnosis, you may want to read *Healing Yourself with Self-Hypnosis,* by Frank Caprio, MD, and Joseph Berger (Prentice Hall Press). You can also read a description of self-hypnosis on the Internet at mentalhelp.net/psyhelp/chap14/chap14w.htm.

Meditating, Doing Yoga, and Praying

Shutting out the world outside and just concentrating on your own inner self or thinking about nothing at all or thinking about a higher power can help you to calm your body down and ease your mind away from the things that bother you so much. It may help you cut back on your painful symptoms of fibromyalgia as well.

Meditation

One of the many forms of meditation may work for you. One study indicated that women with fibromyalgia who practiced daily meditation — about an hour a day for six days a week, over an eight-week period — reported lower levels of pain, better sleep, and lower levels of depression than when they'd begun the study.

Psychologists and other experts can teach methods of meditation, and many communities have free or low-cost classes to provide training on how to meditate. Experts say that meditation is not, however, a quick-fix answer, and the techniques must be learned and practiced for at least a few months before significant results can be noticed.

Yoga

Twisting your body around like a pretzel? Sounds more like a stress-inducing plan instead of something that can cause a state of calmness. So how on earth can yoga help you? Well, first of all, delete the idea from your mind that you must contort your body into impossible positions because that's a stereotypical view of Yoga. True, Yoga does have some very tough positions, but those are for the advanced students, not the beginners.

As with most new forms of exercise, you start slowly and build your way up. When you have fibromyalgia, this building-block policy is particularly important to avoid more strain and pain.

If want to discover much more information on the basics of Yoga — and just about everything else you need to know about this subject — be sure to read *Yoga For Dummies,* by Georg Feuerstein, PhD, and Larry Payne, PhD (published by Wiley).

Prayer

Some people with FMS report that praying helps them feel much better. Prayer may act much in the same way as does meditation or Yoga, instilling calmness and an acceptance that you're really not in control, can't be expected to be accountable for everything, and you need not frantically rush about trying to solve difficult problems right away. Instead, you give yourself a break and (at least temporarily) leave the resolutions of your pain and your problems to the cosmos.

Many churches have "prayer circles," in which you can ask other people to pray for you. You can even find prayer circles on the Internet. In some studies, doctors have found that being prayed for can improve an individual's ability to survive a heart attack or dangerous surgeries. So, why shouldn't they work for fibromyalgia?

Chapter 14

Sweet Dreams! Combating Sleep Disorders

· ·

In This Chapter

▶ Understanding sleep and its importance for people with fibromyalgia

▶ Knowing about sleep stages and their relevance to fibromyalgia syndrome

▶ Discovering common sleep disorders for those with fibromyalgia

▶ Considering lifestyle changes that enhance sleep

▶ Treating sleep disorders with medications and alternative remedies

· ·

*J*uanita's fibromyalgia pain occurs every day, and it's very severe — so bad that she can't work most days and is considering filing for disability bene- fits. Bob's pain is intermittent: some days are overwhelming, and other days he can pretty much ignore the pain and the fatigue. Darlene feels achy and exhausted nearly every day, but she somehow manages to take care of the kids and work part-time.

All three have been diagnosed with fibromyalgia syndrome (FMS), although the severity of their disease and how they cope with it are very different for each person. They all share one common denominator, though: Juanita, Bob, and Darlene have serious sleep problems, each averaging only about four to six hours of sleep nearly every night.

The majority of people with fibromyalgia (at least 75 percent) have sleep diffi- culties, whether they have trouble getting to sleep in the first place or fre- quently wake up after falling asleep. (Some people have both problems.)

Of course, solving sleep disorders doesn't automatically cure your fibromyal- gia. But in many cases, a good night's sleep can considerably ease the pain and the fatigue of your illness. Because pain and fatigue are usually the most troubling symptoms for people with fibromyalgia, resolving sleep problems is clearly very important.

In this chapter, I cover why a good night's sleep is so important for people with fibromyalgia, including spending sufficient quality time in each sleep stage. I also cover the key types of sleep problems that people with FMS experience and offer practical advice on how to achieve the sleep time you need through lifestyle changes, medications, and other immediately doable options.

What is Sleep?

Sleep is a biological process of altered consciousness that all humans must undergo on a regular basis in order to replenish their bodies in physical, biochemical, and psychological ways.

I don't want you to feel like you're in Biology 101, but you do need to have a basic grasp of what exactly *sleep* is and how it affects your body. Sure, you probably think that you *know* what sleep is. It's that process that occurs sometime between going to bed and waking up again. (Or, if you have fibromyalgia, it's that annoying process of trying to rest and waking up with pain and frustration several times each night.) But did you know that sleep has important levels that people need to experience? And did you also know that sleep has necessary biochemical and psychological purposes? Sleep enables the body to repair damaged tissue and also provides the opportunity for dreaming, which scientists have proven is a necessary process for physical and mental health.

Contrary to popular belief, your body doesn't automatically shut down to the point of being just short of switching to the "Off" position when you go to sleep. Some processes slow down, but others speed up. Some important hormones, such as cortisol, growth hormone, and prolactin, are secreted when you sleep or shortly before you wake up. If you don't sleep enough, the production of these hormones can be thrown off, which may increase the probability of pain for fibromyalgia sufferers. Your brain continues to be extremely active in sleep, orchestrating all these processes for you.

Your body also operates with an underlying *circadian rhythm*, like an internal clock for when you're asleep and when you're wide awake. Unfortunately, bad sleep patterns can become engrained sometimes. Don't despair: They can be broken, and I discuss ways to achieve good sleep habits in this chapter.

Understanding the Importance of Sleep Stages

People need to experience enough sleep, in terms of the number of hours that they sleep (usually seven to eight hours per night), and they also need to experience all the different stages of sleep, ranging from light sleep to deep sleep. Some researchers believe that people with fibromyalgia don't spend enough time in the very deep sleep levels. A lack of quality deep sleep may inhibit an adequate production of important protective hormones that are normally made while we sleep, such as growth hormones and *prolactin*. Prolactin is the same hormone that's released by nursing mothers (although sleep releases much less of it), but scientists aren't sure exactly what function prolactin fulfills in nonlactating people.

In 2001, researchers reported on their study of the nighttime hormone levels of women with and without fibromyalgia in the *Journal of Clinical Endocrinology & Metabolism*. They found that women with fibromyalgia (who agreed to take no medication during the study) had significantly lower levels of both nocturnal growth hormone and prolactin. This result provides even more proof that fibromyalgia is real! It also serves as another indicator that people with fibromyalgia should pay special attention to resolving their sleep problems.

Note: Men also release prolactin during deep sleep stages, but less than women.

Here are the three basic types of sleep, according to sleep experts:

✔ Light sleep (Stages 1 and 2)

✔ Deep sleep (Stages 3 and 4)

✔ Rapid eye movement (REM) sleep

Light sleep

Stage 1 is the lightest stage of sleep, and it's also the doorway to eventual dreamland. Many people who are awakened from Stage 1 sleep will deny that they were sleeping at all and may say that they were simply "resting their eyes." In this stage, virtually any little thing — a minor sound or a light touch — can easily awaken the sleeper. In *Stage 2,* another stage of light sleep, you can still wake people up easily, but they'll know that they were asleep if you awaken them then.

Light sleep is important because of its relaxation qualities and also because it's part of the stepwise process that leads to deep sleep and to the rapid eye movement (REM) stage of sleep. You can't get to the deeper stages unless you go through the first two stages of light sleep.

Deep sleep

When you're in the deep and deeper levels of *Stage 3* and *Stage 4* sleep, your body is completely relaxed and people have difficulty waking you up. Stage 4 is also known as *slow-wave* sleep because of the characteristic brain wave patterns of this stage.

During deep sleep, your heart slows down and your breathing becomes regular and relaxed. Your body also releases a small amount of growth hormone, which helps rebuild damaged tissue. Other hormones are also released, such as prolactin and melatonin.

If you don't have enough sleep and, consequently, don't spend enough time in deep sleep, the biochemical processes that are supposed to occur are aborted or may not happen at all. This is probably a key reason why the pain is worse for the FMS sufferer who's slept very little.

If you have trouble sleeping, one tactic that may help is simulating the breathing of a very deep sleep. Doing so may induce your tired body to slip into a sleep state. Try this: Lie down in a comfortable and quiet place. Take in a deep breath and let it out very slowly. Repeat several times. Concentrate only on your breathing and on nothing else. Don't worry about falling asleep, about your fibromyalgia, or work or family problems. Just breathe. Breathing is all that matters.

REM sleep

The REM stage of sleep is the time when dreams occur. This stage is called "rapid eye movement" because scientists have studied the brain waves of people who are dreaming and have noted that sleepers actually move their eyes back and forth under their eyelids at that time, almost as if they were watching a movie. The body may release *cortisol* in this stage (although cortisol can be released anytime during sleep). Cortisol is a hormone released by the adrenal glands. It controls blood pressure, blood sugar, and other key body functions. Some people with FMS may have overly *low* levels of cortisol in the daytime, leading to excessive fatigue, and overly *high* levels at night (causing insomnia). Cortisol production peaks early in the morning, shortly before the sleeper awakes.

Whether dreams have important messages to sleepers is an issue that's been debated for millennia. Some people believe that dreams are like garbage from the brain, akin to the waste material excreted after food is processed by the digestive system. Others believe that dreams hold very important meanings for the dreamer and should be pursued.

I don't know which point of view is right about the significance of dreaming, but I do know that having dreams is important. In experiments in which people were deprived of dreaming (by being wakened when a REM stage was detected), the subjects became very irritable and angry. People with fibromyalgia, like everyone else, need to dream.

When people with fibromyalgia sleep even less than they usually do, they hurt more. Sleep expert William C. Dement, MD, PhD, and Christopher Vaughan say in their book, *The Promise of Sleep* (Dell Trade Paperbacks), that in experiments in which people with fibromyalgia are purposely deprived of sleep, their pain is significantly greater.

Identifying Key Sleep Problems

Everyone has trouble sleeping once in awhile, but suffering from a chronic sleep deficit is a sign of trouble, especially if you have fibromyalgia. For people with FMS, this simple equation is very important: Less sleep = more pain.

In general, people with FMS may have one or all the following sleep difficulties:

- Difficulty falling asleep
- Frequent awakenings
- Lack of deep, restorative sleep

It's 2 a.m. and I'm still awake: Difficulty falling asleep

You've been trying as hard as you can to get yourself to sleep, but your brain just won't cooperate! Instead, it keeps wanting you to think about that problem with the report you were working on today, the bully at school that is harassing your son Johnny, and so many other problems. "Sleep now!" you order yourself — except your body won't cooperate. As you get angrier and more frustrated, the probability of falling asleep soon decreases.

The answer in this situation: Get up, get a drink of water, walk around, and then lie down when you feel like it. Don't be mad at yourself for not falling asleep and don't blame your boss, the nasty kid at school, or anyone else. Be philosophical: these things happen. If insomnia occurs night after night, however, it'll start wearing on your brain and your body, and your fibromyalgia may get worse. Read this chapter carefully and follow my advice.

Too many wake-up calls: You're constantly waking

Another problem many people have is that they fall asleep okay, but they keep waking up. Someone flushes the toilet, and they wake up. They hear a bird chirp, and the sound acts as an untimely wake-up call. It almost seems like a leaf could fall off a tree and wake them up. If you have this problem, you're clearly not getting enough deep sleep.

What can help? For some people, a white noise generator that makes a kind of "SSHHHH" sound can help you tune out that noisy world and fall deeply asleep. Soft music on the radio may help lull you to sleep. Some people can benefit from deep breathing exercises, meditation, or relaxation therapy. (Read Chapter 13 for more information on these techniques.)

Be sure to use the most comfortable mattress that you can find. Sometimes waterbeds are a great solution to help you relax and fall deeply asleep. Some people like cotton flannel sheets because they're cool in the summer and warm in the winter. Check other aspects of your environment as well. For example, is the room too hot or too cold, even if only slightly? If you're uncomfortable, do something to fix the situation and see if that helps you relax.

Insufficient down time in deep sleep

Even when you finally fall asleep, you may spend the night tossing and turning in the early sleep stages and experience an insufficient time in the kind of deep, restorative sleep that your body truly needs. In fact, studies indicate that some people with fibromyalgia suffer from a lack of time in deep sleep.

Lack of exercise can impede sleep

Maybe you haven't been exercising much (or at all) because of your pain and fatigue. But if you could manage some light exercise, such as a short walk an hour or two before bedtime, this activity could help you get to sleep easier. Be sure to read Chapter 15 for more information on how exercising can improve your FMS symptoms.

Understanding sleep apnea

Infrequently, *sleep apnea* is the cause for fatigue or daytime sleepiness. Sleep apnea is a medical problem that causes people (especially people who are overweight) to actually stop breathing while they're asleep. Although each apnea episode lasts for only a short period, and the breathing eventually gets jump-started again by the brain, people can suffer from dozens of these episodes each hour. These lapses of breathing, when added together, can be dangerous for people. In some cases, they can cause heart or lung problems and even be fatal. If your spouse commonly complains that your snoring can be heard in other rooms of the house, or you constantly wake up with choking and coughing, you may have an allergy or a problem with sleep apnea. See your doctor to find out and to receive treatment.

The more you relax (which I know is often not easy!), the more likely you are to achieve a deep, restorative sleep state. Research has shown that, for some people, tricyclic antidepressants, such as Elavil may help to prolong sleep stages 3 and 4. If they don't work, Prozac (generic name: fluoxetine) helps some people. (Read the section, "Taking prescriptions for sleepyland," later in this chapter.)

Analyzing Your Sleep: A Self-test

Answer *True* or *False* to the following eight questions to determine if you or someone you care about may have a sleep problem. And be honest! Nobody but you needs to know your answers.

1. **On most nights, falling asleep takes me an hour or more.**

2. **After I fall asleep, I sleep at least 7 or 8 hours. If I wake up, I fall back to sleep again easily.**

3. **I rely on at least several drinks of beer, wine, or another form of alcohol before bed.**

4. **I consider myself a light sleeper.**

5. **My partner says that I snore.**

6. **When I wake up in the morning, I feel refreshed.**

7. **I take naps on the weekend.**

8. **I like watching scary or exciting TV programs before bed.**

What do your answers mean? Let's take them one by one.

If you answered *True* to the first statement, you have plenty of company — and you also have a sleep problem.

Lisa was diagnosed with fibromyalgia about a year ago, and she says that on most nights, she just lies in bed, and can't sleep. The hours pass from 11 p.m. to 2 a.m., but she still feels almost more wide awake than she did at noon. She wonders what's wrong with her. Part of Lisa's problem may be that she's just trying too hard to fall asleep. Ironically, the harder she tries, the angrier and more frustrated she gets and the less likely she is to fall asleep. Ease up, Lisa! She (and maybe you) needs to try some of the sleep remedies provided later in this chapter.

If you answered *True* to the second statement, good for you! Keep up the good work. Maybe you have some good sleep tips that you can share with your fellow fibromyalgia sufferers.

If you answered *True* to the third statement, you need to break this habit as soon as possible. One glass of beer or wine may be a good way to get to sleep for some people. But more than one glass of beer or wine, as well as drinking any other forms of alcohol, is definitely not a smart choice. You're far more likely to wake up, dehydrated and headachy, around 1 or 2 a.m. with a bad case of insomnia.

If you consider yourself a light sleeper, you may be a person who isn't getting enough sleep. Do you ever feel truly rested in the morning? If not, you need to try my sleep suggestions later in this chapter.

Did you answer *True* to the fifth statement? If so, you may have sleep apnea. Sleep apnea is a dangerous condition by itself. It's also bad because the lack of sleep that this condition induces can also increase the pain of fibromyalgia. Talk to your doctor about resolving this problem.

If you agree with the sixth statement, that you wake up in the morning feeling refreshed, that's great! Sounds like you're doing the right thing. Whatever it is, keep doing it.

If your answer to the seventh statement was *True*, I have to tell you that taking naps on the weekend is a no-no for the person with fibromyalgia — unless a daily siesta is your status quo. If you make naps a weekend-only habit, you may disrupt your sleep cycle. Whenever possible, maintain the same sleep hours (within an hour or two) on weeknights and weekends. You should get up at about the same time every day and go to bed at about the same time every night. This habit is especially important for people with sleep problems — with or without fibromyalgia.

If you become excited or upset by scary or violent movies, as the eighth statement suggests, but you don't want to give them up because you enjoy them, avoid watching them before bedtime. Watch a DVD of *The Mummy Returns* on Saturday afternoon instead of late at night.

Most people don't get enough refreshing sleep, and people with fibromyalgia aren't alone in being sleep deprived. According to a survey performed by the National Sleep Foundation in 2000, two-thirds of 1,000 people reported having trouble sleeping at least a few times a week. In fact, sometimes the sleep deprivation is voluntary. Nearly half (45 percent) said that they'd sacrifice more sleep if they could get more done. Yet sleep deprivation leads to car crashes, mistakes at work, and yelling at your kids. A good night's sleep is important for everyone, and it's especially vital for people with FMS.

Adjusting Your Lifestyle to Cope with the Problem

Medications can help you fall asleep and sleep peacefully through the night, and I discuss drugs in the next section. But you can also make simple changes in your life that will often help carry you off into the wonderful world of sleep. The following are some good lifestyle options:

- ✔ Pay attention to what you eat and drink at dinnertime and afterwards.

- ✔ Discover how to relax (Read more about relaxation therapy in Chapter 10).

- ✔ Accept that your bed is for sleeping only (Okay, it's for sex, too. But that's it!). Do your working, reading, and TV watching elsewhere.

- ✔ Encourage a snoring partner to get help. If he or she refuses to get help, consider using earplugs or a white noise machine to help cancel out the noise.

Consuming soporific suppers

If you suffer from insomnia, you should avoid eating a fashionably late dinner (after 8 p.m.) and also be sure to take other basic steps that can facilitate sleep. For example, avoid all caffeine (coffee, tea, cola drinks, and chocolate) after 5 p.m., so your system won't be overstimulated when it's time to fall asleep. Consider eating foods that are known to be rich in natural tryptophan, a chemical that induces sleep. Turkey's packed with it. Milk also has this substance, although in lower quantities.

Eating a few pieces of turkey or a turkey sandwich, combined with a glass of milk, an hour before when you want to go to sleep may relax you enough to help you nod off without (or with less) difficulty. Of course, you shouldn't overeat, which can defeat your purpose because you may get a stomachache and find it even more difficult to fall asleep.

Relaxing

Falling asleep is nearly impossible when your body is tense from the day's battles and problems. But you can discover how to relax, whether through deep breathing (discussed in this chapter), relaxation therapy (see Chapter 10) or through special relaxing exercises, such as Chinese T'ai Chi (refer to Chapter 12). The point is, relaxation isn't bad; it's absolutely necessary. Yet in our achievement-oriented society, where many people think every nanosecond must be a productive one, relaxation may be a tough concept to accept as being good.

Think of it this way: even machines need some "down" time. Your body is a wonderful and unique kind of biological machine, and it definitely needs some time off from intensive efforts. And it needs that time off every day. It needs restorative sleep. And besides, good sleep can enable *more* productivity the next day. Don't deny yourself this important need.

Using your bed for sleeping (and sex)

Your bed is for sleeping. This statement may sound obvious, but too many people don't grasp this simple point. Your bed really isn't a good place to read books, grade papers, or perform other nonrestful activities. With the exception of sexual activities (which are also good for your body and may help you sleep deeply), do nothing in your bed except sleep. Perform your other activities elsewhere.

Quieting a snoring partner

What if you're not the one who's snoring, but rather your partner is? Encourage him or her to get help. Your partner may have sleep apnea, a sinus infection, or some other medical problem. The snoring is also disrupting your sleep! Resolving this snoring problem can help you both.

Slipping Into Slumber Using Medications and Other Remedies

Sometimes, you try lifestyle changes, limit your heavy meals, and follow my other good suggestions in this chapter and this book, but you're still not registering enough "Zs." You may need to try a sleep medication. Over-the-counter medicines, alternative remedies, and prescribed medicines are all available today and just may help you.

Buying nonprescription medicines

You can purchase over-the-counter sleep remedies at your pharmacy or even your supermarket. Most of these drugs have the same ingredients as antihistamines (cold and allergy medicines). They may make you a little drowsy, but generally, they have a limited effectiveness at inducing sleep. In most cases when they do induce sleep, these medications fail to deliver significant restorative sleep to their users. They can cause constipation, dry mouth, and other side effects. They may also cause *rebound insomnia,* which means that these medicines actually cause you to have insomnia if you stop taking the medicine. If you have insomnia, you need a sleep remedy, not an allergy drug.

If you do decide to use an over-the-counter sleep remedy, be sure to read the instructions on the package and any inserts first. You don't want to risk having the drug interact with other medications you may be taking for fibromyalgia or other illnesses you have. If possible, ask your doctor if he or she recommends this medicine or considers it safe. You can also call the doctor's office and ask the nurse to ask the physician for you.

Using helpful alternative remedies

Alternative remedies to the standard over-the-counter medications are effective in helping some people get to sleep. Some key alternative remedies are *valerian, kava kava, and melatonin.*

Letting your doctor know that you plan to take or are already taking herbal medicines or other supplements is very important. These alternative remedies can interact with other medicines you're taking.

Valerian

Clinical studies in the United States, the United Kingdom, and Germany on the use of valerian as a mild sedative have proven that this herbal root does help some people with their insomnia. Studies also indicate that valerian doesn't appear to affect sleep stages negatively or to impede the concentration or reactions of users on the day after they use it.

According to the American Society of Anesthesiologists, valerian may boost the effects of some antiseizure medicines. If you take an antiseizure medicine, be sure to ask your doctor if you can safely take valerian. Better yet, try a different remedy.

Kava kava

What about the herbal remedy kava kava? This herb (also known as *Piper methysticum*) has been used by people for problems of insomnia, stress, anxiety, and premenstrual syndrome. In a study reported in *Phytotherapy Research* in 2001, researchers treated subjects who suffered from stress-induced insomnia with kava kava for several weeks and then treated them with valerian. The researchers found that both herbs were effective. The most frequent side effect found with valerian was vivid dreams, experienced by 16 percent of the subjects. The most frequent side effect experienced with kava kava was dizziness, experienced by 12 percent of the subjects.

In late 2001, the Food and Drug Administration (FDA) issued a warning that some people in Europe who've used kava kava have experienced severe liver toxicity (damage to the liver, a crucial organ that you can't live without), suffering from such problems as hepatitis, cirrhosis, and even liver failure. In addition, the FDA also received reports on Americans experiencing liver problems with taking kava kava.

Melatonin

The hormone melatonin has proven effective at helping some people get to sleep, and studies indicate that melatonin may be especially helpful for travelers who are plagued with problems of jet lag. The drug appears to reset the natural body rhythm of the user. Your body actually produces melatonin naturally (it's produced by the pineal gland in your brain). But you may need an extra boost from nature from time to time, and taking supplemental melatonin may help you. Keep in mind, however, that melatonin has been reported to cause headaches, stomachaches, strange dreams, and even depression in some people.

Taking prescriptions for sleepyland

Are prescribed medications for sleep safe? In most cases, *yes,* although you should pay attention to your doctor's warnings about side effects, the dose you should take, and any other warnings your doctor gives you. Also ask your pharmacist about any side effects or potential interactions with other medications you're taking.

The key medications that are prescribed to help people sleep are:

- ✔ Ambien (generic name: zolpidem)
- ✔ Antidepressant medications
- ✔ Fibromyalgia medications that also induce sleep

Ambien

Approved by the FDA in 1992, Ambien is the most popular prescribed drug for insomniacs in the United States. It also appears to have few side effects. Ambien doesn't cause people to have a "drugged-out" or stuporous feeling in the morning. A very small percentage (about 1 to 2 percent) of Ambien users have problems with continued daytime drowsiness, dizziness, and diarrhea.

Don't take sedating medications during daylight hours unless you can stay home. Don't even think about driving a car or operating any type of equipment beyond perhaps turning on your computer.

Antidepressants

Doctors frequently prescribe antidepressant medications for people with fibromyalgia. These drugs are not usually prescribed in a high enough dose to treat someone with depression, but instead, doctors order them at a lower dose to help induce sleep and also to ease pain from fibromyalgia or other medical problems.

Drugs, such as Elavil (generic name: amitriptyline) and Desyrel (generic name: trazodone) make most people tired, and they fall asleep. The downside is that these drugs may also cause weight gain and a "druggy" feeling the next day in some people. Dry eyes and mouth are other side effects that can occur.

Prozac (generic name: fluoxetine) may help some people achieve a deeper sleep if other antidepressants don't work well. One rather unfortunate side effect is that Prozac may inhibit orgasm in some people.

Other sleep-inducing medications

Some pain medications that doctors prescribe for people with fibromyalgia also induce sedation, so doctors may feel that they're conquering two problems with one drug. (Read more on medications in Chapter 13.) Flexeril (generic name: cyclobenzaprine) is a muscle relaxant that makes many users feel drowsy. Ultram (generic name: tramadol) is another effective pain medication that also has sedating effects.

Most patients take these drugs at night because of their sedative effects, even when the medications are taken primarily to control pain. If they're taken during the day, patients must usually refrain from performing tasks that require high alertness.

Chapter 15

Exercising, Losing Weight, and Avoiding Trigger Foods/Drinks

. . . .

In This Chapter

▶ Exercising and how it can improve how you feel

▶ Working on weight loss to decrease pain

▶ Staying away from foods that may worsen your pain

. . . .

*Y*ou've heard it all before: You should exercise, lose weight, and do all that boring and hard stuff that most doctors constantly urge so many of their patients to do. But the reality is — they're right!

Exercising and losing weight (if you're overweight) really *can* help you feel better by decreasing your fibromyalgia pain, fatigue, and muscle stiffness. And here's a little secret: You don't have to exercise to the point of exhaustion, nor do you have to lose great amounts of weight to feel better.

This chapter talks about several important lifestyle changes that you can make to gain more control over your fibromyalgia syndrome (FMS) symptoms. First, I cover the benefits of exercising. I also include some basic do's and don'ts on exercising and provide four simple exercises for you to try. Next, I cover weight loss, providing you with a chart to determine for yourself whether you need to lose weight. I also cover several popular prescribed diet drugs and their basic pros and cons.

Finally, I cover dietary "excitotoxins," a made-up word that connotes food substances that some experts believe can aggravate your FMS symptoms. You may just find that avoiding these substances will help to improve your condition.

Exercising to Relieve FMS Pain

Most people associate painkilling with a variety of over-the-counter or pre-scribed medications. But drugs aren't the only means to improving your fibromyalgia symptoms. Getting "physical" by starting a plan of exercising can work well, too, although exercising may seem like a sort of strange way to gain pain relief. Gentle, low-stress, paced exercising can make you feel better, loosening your muscles and greasing your stiff joints now and possibly acting as a preventive measure to ease your pain down the road.

Some studies have indicated that people with fibromyalgia have a basic fitness level that's significantly lower than the levels that are found among people who don't have fibromyalgia. (Not that amazing after you think about it because people with FMS generally feel pretty bad, and thus, they're less likely to be physically fit.) Regular exercise may help people with FMS to close that gap, but it won't happen in just a few days or even in a few weeks. Be patient and persistent, and you'll get there.

Here are a few tips to keep in mind as you gear up to exercise:

✔ **Create a basic fitness program that suits your needs.** Realize also that if you were more athletic in the past, as many people with fibromyalgia report that they were, that was *then*. Make a plan that works for you and your needs as they are *now*.

✔ **Set a realistic goal.** Whether exercise goals are set by a physician, a physical therapist, a personal trainer, or anyone else (including you), the goals for a person with fibromyalgia shouldn't be the same as for a person who doesn't have fibromyalgia because people with FMS have a lower pain tolerance and tire faster than others. Too much exercise, too fast, can accelerate their pain. Physical expectations need to be scaled down considerably for the person who has FMS.

✔ **Consult with your physician before you start your new exercise program.** Run your plan by your physician. She may want to check out your overall fitness level with a treadmill test or with other screening measures. She may also merely listen to your plan, nod wisely, and then give you the thumbs up, wishing you well.

✔ **Start slowly and steadily build your way up.** Start with just five minutes a day for several times a week (except for walking, which can be for longer periods). Then every four to five days or so, add on another minute of exercise. Keep adding on minutes, until you're up to about a half-hour for three to four days per week. You can also increase the speed at which you perform your exercises, gauging how fast to go by your own comfort level.

Note: When it comes to walking, many people with FMS should be able to follow the walking program in the chart in this chapter, walking up to 60 minutes after 12 weeks. Walking is a good exercise, but it's a moderate, steady type of exercise; thus, you can walk for a longer period than you can perform reps of strenuous exercises.

✔ **Keep it simple.** Consider the simple exercises offered in this chapter, which can help you build up your strength and cut back on your pain level without breaking your bank on expensive gym memberships or personal trainers.

✔ **Don't overdo it!** Now isn't the time to adopt "No pain, no gain!" as your prevailing motto. It simply doesn't work for people who have fibromyalgia. A little discomfort is okay and sweating is good. But actual pain? Forgettaboutit.

Prepare for exercising by drinking plenty of fluids and making sure that you dress comfortably and appropriately. Skip the spandex pants and tight t-shirts. Wear something loose fitting. If you plan to exercise outside and the weather seems iffy or you're not sure whether it's going to be cold or moderate, wear a few layers of clothes, such as a shirt and a sweatshirt and pants. You can always take the sweatshirt off if you get too warm. Be sure that you wear good, comfortable walking shoes. Don't worry about the fashion police. Assume that they've taken the day off.

Exploring Pain-Relieving Exercises

An effective exercise designed to alleviate pain over time is simple to perform and doesn't take a lot of time, and yet it adequately manipulates the targeted muscle groups. Here are a few ideas for you to try.

Walking off the pain and strain of FMS

Walking is an excellent and easy exercise for most people, and it's one that most can perform nearly every day. It doesn't cost anything, and you decide when the time is right and where you want to walk.

However, when you feel really bad, even walking can be hard to do, and it may cause you some pain. So you shouldn't strive for long distances — at least when you first start your walking program. And don't strain yourself to keep up with others who may be in much more of a rush than you are. Pace yourself. Walk briskly, but don't push too hard. You know how fast is fast enough for you.

Table 15-1 shows a walking program for you to try, developed by the United States federal government. It allows you to build up slowly. Use the program as is or adapt it to your needs. During the warmup portion, walk at a comfortable pace and work up to a brisk pace for the exercise portion. When you're ready for the cool-down, begin walking at a slower pace to get your heart rate back down.

Table 15-1	A Sample Walking Program			
Week Number	**Warmup**	**Exercising**	**Cool-down**	**Total Time**
1	5 min.	5 min.	5 min.	15 min.
2	5 min.	7 min.	5 min.	17min.
3	5 min.	9 min.	5 min.	19 min.
4	5min.	11 min.	5 min.	21 min.
5	5 min.	13 min.	5 min.	23 min.
6	5 min.	15 min.	5 min.	25 min.
7	5 min.	18 min.	5 min.	28 min.
8	5 min.	20 min.	5 min.	30 min.
9	5 min.	23 min.	5 min.	33 min.
10	5 min.	26 min.	5 min.	36 min.
11	5 min.	28 min.	5 min.	38 min.
12	5 min.	30 min.	5 min.	40 min.

After you complete Week 12, gradually increase your brisk walking time to 60 minutes, 3 or 4 times a week.

TIP

Make your walk fun and enjoyable by walking with your spouse or a friend or taking your dog on some extra walks. (Or get a dog, so you can take it for walks!) Music can make exercising easier and much more fun as well. Play your favorite music while you perform the exercises described in this chapter or other exercises that you and your doctor have identified as helpful. Headphones make it simple for you to eliminate the teasing you may receive from your family members or others for listening to Elvis, Britney Spears, Aretha, or whatever other type of music that *you* like. Go for upbeat, energetic music, whether it's pop, show tunes, or whatever.

After you've become used to walking, you'll probably actually miss your daily walk if you have to forego it due to bad weather or some other circumstance. (No kidding! You'll actually start to look forward to your daily workouts.) So, you may want a plan for walking indoors when the need arises. If bad weather or long work hours prevent you from walking outside, drive to the nearest shopping mall and walk several laps around the entire mall.

You should also incorporate more walking into other parts in your daily life. For example, when you go shopping at the supermarket or elsewhere, don't consider it a major victory when you can park practically next to the front door entrance. Instead, park farther away and then walk a little farther than usual. A side benefit of parking farther away is you won't have other drivers lined up and eager to take your very close spot, trying to hustle you out of there. When you're out in "left field," you can take your time to reach your car, find your car keys, and get yourself comfortable, and nobody will care.

When you need to enter a building that's a few stories high, ignore the elevator and take the stairs instead. It's great exercise for your heart as well as the rest of your body. Don't run up the stairs: Take your time.

Be sure that you move around and change positions frequently in your daily life. Sure, the movie is fascinating, or maybe another project that you're working on has you mesmerized. You may feel like (or act as if) you're "glued" to your chair. If so, unstick yourself. At least every 15 to 20 minutes, get up and move around. And then, if you want, return to the previously intriguing activity. Moving around more frequently can help abate some of the muscle stiffness that's so common for people with fibromyalgia.

Swimming, cycling, and other choices

Swimming, cycling, and strengthening exercises are good for your muscles, your heart, and your whole body. Getting into shape can be a very effective preventive tactic, helping to shield you against future pain and fatigue. You can't get a brand new body (not yet, anyway!). But you can and should work on strengthening the one you have.

Analyzing aquatic exercises: Water works

Aquatic exercises range from making simple movements in the pool all the way up to swimming laps. So the range of activity choices is considerable. Aquatic exercises are easier on the body than are exercises performed out of the water because water exerts less strain and "drag" on the body and allows for a greater freedom of movement. (Less strain and more movement are great selling points for people with FMS.)

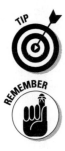

One very simple water exercise is to walk around in the shallow end of the pool. Keep your arms under the water line, so they don't create too much pull and strain on your body.

If you exercise in a swimming pool, the water should be comfortably warm because many people with fibromyalgia are very sensitive to cold temperatures and find it harder to move when they're immersed in cold (or hot) water. Always check the temperature of the water with a pool thermometer before jumping in. Some experts recommend that the water temperature should be set between 83° and 90° F. If you use a public pool, ask the staff whether they have a pool thermometer you can borrow to test the temperature because you're highly sensitive to heat and cold. You can also buy a pool thermometer for a few dollars in a pool supply store.

If you want to take a local class in water aerobics in a warm water pool, check your local newspaper for further information or contact your local chapter of the Arthritis Foundation to find out information on dates and times of classes that are offered. If you're not sure how to find your local chapter, call the national Arthritis Foundation toll free at 800-283-7800 or check their Web site (www.arthritis.org).

Cycling to symptom reduction

Riding your bike is also a great exercise, even if it's just around the block. Or you can use a stationary bike and cycle yourself ahead many "miles" while you stay in your home and watch Oprah, a PBS program, or your favorite movie, or while you listen to music or an audiotape of a book.

Getting stronger with strengthening exercises

If you begin practicing strengthening exercises, you can build your body up and make it more impervious to pain. However, avoid weightlifting because that may increase your pain. With little or no exercising, you're like a weak new tiger cub. With regular exercising, you may not make it all the way to a strong tigress. But you'll be a lot closer.

The exercise shown in Figure 15-1 helps you strengthen your upper back and shoulder muscles, often major problem areas for many people with fibromyalgia.

1. **Assume a hands-and-knees position on your exercise mat (don't do this exercise on the hard floor with no mat!) with your neck straight and parallel to the floor.**

2. **Slowly stretch your right arm out in front of you, keeping your arm straight and parallel to the floor, to about the height of your ear. (Your fingers should point at the wall on the opposite side of the room and should be together.)**

3. **Hold this position for five seconds, if possible. Then slowly return your arm to its starting position.**

4. **Repeat the exercise with your other arm and then alternate. Try for ten repetitions, if you can manage that many comfortably.**

Figure 15-1:
Shoulder arm extension. This will help your upper back and can also improve your posture as well.

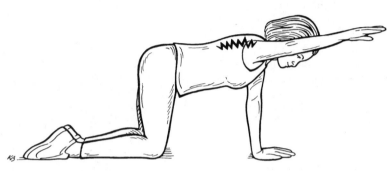

The exercise shown in Figure 15-2 is effective at toning both your side and back muscles and can be effective in preventing sudden back spasms that may result from turning or twisting the wrong way.

1. **Stand up straight with your feet about 18 inches apart.**

2. **Bend your left elbow and place your left hand at your waist akimbo, as depicted.**

3. **Straighten your right arm over your head while, at the same time, trying to keep your right shoulder level with the left shoulder.**

4. **Bend slowly toward the left (toward your bent elbow), keeping your right arm above your head. Feel the pull in your right side. Hold this position for the count of five. (Don't push your right hip to the side as you bend. That can put extra stress on your knees. It's also cheating.)**

5. **Slowly return to an upright position.**

6. **Repeat on the other side. Try for ten repetitions on each side.**

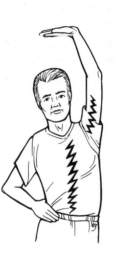

Figure 15-2:
Side stretch. Stretching is important in fibro-myalgia, and this exercise will help by stretching the muscles that extend from your upper arm to your hip.

The exercise shown in Figure 15-3 is really good for tightening your abdominal muscles, the ones that support your lower back. The mini sit-up causes your abdominals to contract and to hold at the point of maximum resistance, without overly straining your back and neck muscles.

1. **Lie flat on your back on your exercise mat. Bend your knees, keeping your feet flat on the floor. (Your knees should be no more than an inch or two apart.)**

2. **Fold your arms across your chest and raise your head, neck, and shoulders off the floor. Your head and neck will curl forward, but they shouldn't curl forward enough to cause your chin to be on your chest.**

3. **Hold this position for a count of five. Suck in your stomach muscles as you do this.**

4. **Slowly release, and roll back down to your starting position.**

5. **Repeat this exercise five times, if possible.**

The exercise shown in Figure 15-4 will loosen up your hip joint while, at the same time, stretching your lower back and buttock muscles.

1. **Lie on your back on your exercise mat, legs extended and arms at your sides.**

2. Bend your right leg, grab it with both hands just below the knee, and pull it gently towards your chest as far as you can.

3. Hold your leg at this maximum position for a count of five, making sure that your other leg is straight and on the floor.

4. Slowly release and repeat the exercise with your left leg. Try for ten repetitions on each leg, if possible.

Figure 15-3:
Mini sit-up. This simple exercise will tighten your abdominal muscles while avoiding placing stress on your back and neck.

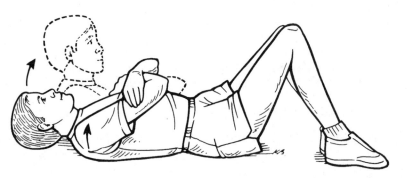

Figure 15-4:
Knee to chest stretch. This stretching exercise is excellent for the lower back, buttock muscles, and your hip joint.

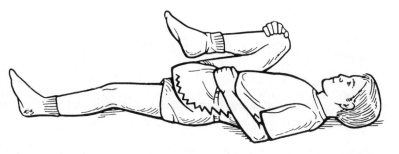

Losing Weight to Decrease Pain and Fatigue

If you happen to be carrying around some extra pounds on you (or maybe a lot of extra weight), this problem isn't actually causing your fibromyalgia. However, the additional weight can and usually does worsen the already-existing condition. Conversely, dropping a few pounds can make you feel significantly better. You don't have to lose an enormous amount of poundage. You'll feel and look better as soon as you lose the first few pounds, which can motivate you to continue to lose weight at a slow and healthy pace until you reach your ideal weight.

Not only will weight loss improve (although not eliminate) your fibromyalgia symptoms, but weight loss (if you're overweight) will also decrease your risk for developing diabetes, hypertension, and many other health problems that are directly associated with obesity.

Give yourself small, doable goals. Even if you need to lose a lot of weight, shoot for 3 or 4 pounds as your initial goal. When you do lose your initial target goal of 3 or 4 pounds, reward yourself (but not with food!). Give yourself a small but nice bonus — maybe buy yourself a new outfit or hit the town for a night of dancing. Then give yourself a few days or weeks to maintain that weight and, when you feel ready, set a new goal to lose another small amount of weight. Each time you reach your new goal, praise yourself lavishly in your mind. Focus on what you've achieved by losing those 3 or 4 pounds at each new level.

Figuring your ideal weight

How much should you weigh? The United States federal government has devised its own unisex tables of *body mass index* (BMI), a height/weight measure. This information provides some basic guidance on how much weight is too low, just right, and over the top for your height.

You can easily determine your current body mass index by checking Table 15-2, a table of BMI levels provided by the federal government. The BMI is derived from a rather complicated formula, but you don't have to drag out your calculator or your old high school math book to do the equations. The nice people who made the chart have already done all those calculations for you.

Find out where you fit on the BMI chart, based on your height and weight. Then review Table 15-3, "Body Mass Index Classification," to see where you fit. In general, if your body mass index is 30 or greater, you're considered to be carrying around too many pounds.

Table 15-2						Body Mass Index Chart								
Body Mass Index (kg/m^2)														
	19	20	21	22	23	24	25	26	27	28	29	30	35	40
Height (inches/ meters)	**Body Weight (pounds)**													
58/1.47	91	96	100	105	110	115	119	124	129	134	138	143	167	191
59/1.50	94	99	104	109	114	119	124	128	133	138	143	148	173	198
60/1.52	97	102	107	112	118	123	128	133	138	143	148	153	179	204
61/1.55	100	106	111	116	122	127	132	137	143	148	153	158	185	211
62/1.57	104	109	115	120	126	131	136	142	147	153	158	164	191	218
63/1.60	107	113	118	124	130	135	141	146	152	158	163	169	197	225
64/1.63	110	116	122	128	134	140	145	151	157	163	169	174	204	232
65/1.65	114	120	126	132	138	144	150	156	162	168	174	180	210	240
66/1.68	118	124	130	136	142	148	155	161	167	173	179	186	216	247
67/1.70	121	127	134	140	146	153	159	166	172	178	185	191	223	255
68/1.73	125	131	138	144	151	158	164	171	177	184	190	197	230	262
69/1.75	128	135	142	149	155	162	169	176	182	189	196	203	236	270
70/1.78	132	139	146	153	160	167	174	181	188	195	202	207	243	278
71/1.80	136	143	150	157	165	172	179	186	193	200	208	215	250	286
72/1.83	140	147	154	162	169	177	184	191	199	206	213	221	258	294
73/1.85	144	151	159	166	174	182	189	197	204	212	219	227	265	302
74/1.88	148	155	163	171	179	186	194	202	210	218	225	233	272	311
75/1.90	152	160	168	176	184	192	200	208	216	224	232	240	279	319
76/1.93	156	164	172	180	189	197	205	213	221	230	238	246	287	328

Table 15-3 provides the classifications for adults, according to the National Heart, Lung, and Blood Institute.

Table 15-3: Body Mass Index Levels

Body Mass Index Classification	BMI
Underweight	Less than 18.5
Normal weight	18.5-24.9
Overweight	25-29.9
Obesity (class 1)	30-34.9
Obesity (class 2)	35-39.9
Extreme obesity	40 or over

For example, suppose that Mary Sunshine is 5 feet 4 inches (or 64 inches), and she weighs 174 pounds. Her BMI is 31, which means that Mary is categorized within "Class 1," the lower end of the "obesity" scale. To move downward into the "overweight" category — which still isn't "normal," but is better than obese — Mary would need to drop down to just 169 pounds, a mere five -pound weight loss.

If Mary then decides that she wants to catapult herself all the way into the "normal" range, she would need to shoot for weighing about 140 pounds. Ms. Sunshine shouldn't even think about, however, trying to drop down to the weight of most TV stars or models. No, no, Mary, bad plan! Many celebrities have a BMI that is very unhealthy and very underweight. Mary Sunshine wants to be (or should want to be) in the normal and healthy range. As should *you*.

Improving your diet and exercising to shed pounds

Weight loss medications exist for people who simply can't get the pounds off, no matter what they do. But before you resort to prescribed medications and their side effects, you need to work on exercising and changing your diet. I know, I know, it sounds boring and a lot harder than popping a pill. But for most people, it's the best way.

Exercise is good, but you should be sure to pace yourself. Because fibromyalgia is a condition with frequent ups and downs, you may make the mistake of demanding too much of yourself on those days when you're feeling better.

Many people associate food with certain behaviors. Change the behavior, and you can help yourself lose weight. For example, if the coffee machine at work always has plenty of sweets and other "goodies" around it, go get your coffee and leave fast. Or better yet, bring water to work, and you won't even have to look at the junk food and then have to make a conscious decision to not eat it. Another idea: Instead of meeting your friends for lunch at a restaurant, where you just sit and eat, meet them instead at a museum or a park and spend the time walking around and chatting with each other. Bring a nutritious picnic lunch for eating outside and enjoy!

Eat slowly and use smaller plates. If you chew your food more slowly, savoring it (but not so slowly that it becomes tasteless and disgusting), you give your brain appetite centers time to kick in and tell you, "Stop! I'm full!" If you rush your eating, you're more likely to overeat because your appetite center hasn't had a chance to react. Using smaller plates may sound silly, but experts say that it does work. Smaller portions don't look so small on smaller plates.

Considering some weight loss meds

What if you've tried really, really hard to lose weight and have increased your exercise, but you've gotten nowhere? Those pounds keep hanging on to you like iron filings to a magnet.

Would making use of weight loss drugs help you drop some of those pounds? Possibly, although you should consider some pros and cons to their use before you start taking them. In addition, you should realize that, despite the dramatic advertising hype you may read about or see on television, none of them are miracle drugs.

Many different weight loss medications are on the market today. Some can be bought in your local supermarket or pharmacy and others require a prescription.

I generally don't recommend over-the-counter weight loss meds, despite their wonderful-sounding promises and the startling "before" and "after" pictures. The reality is that over-the-counter weight loss remedies don't work for most people, and some remedies (such as some herbal remedies) can be dangerous or fatal. Also, in most cases, as soon as you *stop* taking an over-the-counter drug for weight loss, the pounds usually pile back on.

As for prescribed medications, the two most popular are *Xenical* (generic name: orlistat) and *Meridia* (generic name: sibutramine.) These two drugs work in different ways to help people lose weight and are usually only recommended for obese people, and not for those who need to lose just a few pounds.

Prescribed medications may cause some aggravating side effects, such as high blood pressure and even fecal leakage. Also, you may need to take prescribed weight loss medicines indefinitely, although their long-term effects of more than a year have not been tested so far. And even after taking the medication for a long period of time, you may experience weight gain after you *stop* taking the medication. Be sure to talk frankly with your doctor about prescribed weight loss medications before you begin taking one, and be sure to discontinue the use of any over-the-counter weight loss remedies while taking prescription weight loss meds.

People who need to lose only 3 to 5 pounds should never use weight loss medicines of any kind. Remember, your weight fluctuates. Some people may weigh themselves at night, and the next morning, their weight could have changed by as much as 3 pounds.

Researchers are working hard on developing and testing new medications that may enable people to lose a great deal of weight in the near future, but these drugs are still in the clinical testing stage. They'll probably not be introduced to the general public for at least four or five years, at the earliest. These drugs seem to work well on laboratory rats, but it'll take time before researchers know whether they're safe and effective when people use them.

Discovering Dietary Effects: Good Foods/Bad Foods

You probably can't alleviate your fibromyalgia entirely by watching what you eat. However, studies have indicated that you may be able to reduce your pain level and even improve your quantity and quality of sleep by plotting a course toward certain foods and away from others.

People with FMS are different from each other, and no large-scale studies have found that some foods are good and others should be banned for people with fibromyalgia, but some patterns are beginning to emerge. For example, some fibromyalgia sufferers agree that most fruits and vegetables (especially berries) and plain cereals are FMS-friendly, but chocolate; citrus fruits; and foods high in *monosodium glutamate* (MSG), a chemical that's regarded as a "flavor enhancer;" *aspartame,* an artificial sweetener; or caffeine aggravate their FMS symptoms. Check food labels to see whether MSG or aspartame is included in the product. (Just so you know, you may have a harder time giving up aspartame because it's found in a wide variety of products, particularly diet soft drinks and reduced-calorie foods.)

If you find that MSG gives you trouble, when you eat out in restaurants, consider telling the waiter that you're allergic to MSG, and it should not be added to your food. (You can also simply request that MSG not be added to your food, but that request may be ignored. If you say that you're *allergic,* your request is more likely to be heeded. It's not entirely a falsehood, either, because MSG *can* cause a flare-up of FMS symptoms.)

As for beverages, plain old water is best to drink. You may think that water is really boring — but have you checked the water aisle of your supermarket lately? You can get water with lemon or other flavors added, and you can get carbonated water if you like bubbles. If you don't want fancy water, local tap water will work just fine.

One way to figure out whether specific foods make your symptoms worse is to keep a food diary. Each day, write down everything you eat on one side of a sheet of paper. On the other side of your paper (and at the end of the day), list any symptoms that are worse than usual, such as worsened pain or greater fatigue. Keep your food diary for at least two weeks and compare what you ate with how you felt. If you notice that you felt worse on those days when you ate ice cream and milk and had whipped cream on your pie, maybe dairy products are a problem for you. If you felt bad when you ate some pecan pie, maybe nuts bother you. If you start to see a pattern, try eliminating the suspicious food for at least a week or two and notice if you feel any different. If you feel better without it, that food may be a problem for you and should go on your "avoid" list.

Chapter 16

Coping with Emotions: Your Own

● ●

In This Chapter

▶ Understanding what depression is and how to deal with it

▶ Feeling anxious: what to do

▶ Taking your emotional temperature: a self-test

▶ Finding a therapist if you need one

▶ Thinking about medications for emotional problems

● ●

*F*ibromyalgia can be so painful, and its symptoms so distressing that the illness may drive people who have it into depression or anxiety. The existence of an emotional problem occurs frequently with chronic illness, and fibromyalgia syndrome (FMS) is no exception. Depression and/or anxiety can worsen pain and other symptoms of fibromyalgia. Some studies indicate that many people with fibromyalgia respond to their illness with resignation and passivity. But confronting emotional difficulties and seeking help usually work much better than denying them or hoping that they'll go away.

In this chapter, I cover the most common emotional problems faced by people with fibromyalgia. At the top of my list is depression because people with fibromyalgia often experience this problem. I help you identify the basic symptoms of this common illness, and I also offer advice on how to work on resolving depression. Anxiety is another common problem among people with fibromyalgia, as is stress. (I cover stress and "de-stressing" yourself in Chapter 13.) This chapter focuses on anxiety's general manifestations among people with FMS and provides practical advice on what to do if anxiety is overwhelming you.

You may have trouble knowing exactly *what* your emotional status actually is, especially if you've been feeling very bad for a long time. People often become emotionally numbed by their personal problems, as well as by their chronic pain. So I offer a self-test to take your "emotional temperature," and I explain what your answers may mean and what you should do about them. I also talk about how to find a good therapist, and I cover the primary psychiatric medications prescribed by doctors when you're diagnosed with depression or anxiety. "All that in one chapter?" you ask. I aim to please.

Dealing with Depression

Depression is far more widespread than most people realize, and many people will experience clinical depression at some point in their lives — whether they have fibromyalgia or not. But people suffering from fibromyalgia are particularly vulnerable to this illness.

Defining depression and its symptoms

Depression is an extreme form of sadness, which manifests itself in feelings of continued and severe hopelessness or helplessness. People throw the word around a lot to denote having a bad day or feeling a little sad, but depression is much more complicated than that. Depression is a mood disorder that lasts longer than a few days or even a few weeks. It's not something that people can talk themselves out of, nor can others cheer them up from it.

Depression manifests itself differently in different people. Some people cry constantly when depressed; others constantly yell at everyone else or behave aggressively. Here are some symptoms of a possible depression:

- A recent dramatic decrease or increase in appetite, causing a weight change of ten or more pounds in a month
- Frequent thoughts of suicide and/or a plan for suicide
- Lack of interest in activities that were considered captivating in the past
- A dramatic drop in energy and activity levels
- Extreme guilt
- A continued sense of hopelessness
- Excessive agitation or anger
- Sleeping excessively, or difficulty sleeping

If you have any of these symptoms, you should see your doctor or a therapist. Read my section on taking your emotional temperature for further insights.

Connecting FMS and clinical depression

Probably the majority of people with fibromyalgia suffer from some level of chronic depression. Which came first — the fibromyalgia or the depression — isn't always clear. Maybe they both seemed to appear at about the same time. But *when* the depression appeared isn't all that important. What's important is identifying depression when it *does* appear and working to control it. Physicians say that depression is one of the most treatable medical problems around. But it's not going to get better on its own. It requires some work.

Treating depression

Linda says that she stopped listening to her children and her husband, and she spent most of her days in a fog of despair and hopelessness. She couldn't work anymore, so she stayed home — but she's not really sure what happened during those days. The pain and fatigue from the fibromyalgia, combined with her depression, made life almost unbearable. Linda's husband recognized that his wife was in a dangerous state, and he insisted that she see a psychiatrist. Linda was so apathetic that she agreed.

The doctor quickly diagnosed depression and placed Linda on Zoloft (generic name: sertraline), an antidepressant. He also recommended that Linda start a daily walking program, and he urged her to go to a pain specialist to get her pain under control. Within a few weeks of following the doctor's orders, and also seeing a rheumatologist experienced at treating FMS, Linda's depression began to lift, her pain levels dropped, and she began to believe that she could manage this fibromyalgia thing. She went back to work part-time and hopes to eventually work up to full-time work.

Unfortunately, depression isn't always so easily treated. Many people also need to talk about their emotional problems with a trained professional, such as a psychiatrist or a psychologist, to gain some resolution. And, sometimes, several different medications have to be tried (one after the other). Much more than your primary care physician, psychiatrists are best equipped to prescribe antidepressants and other drugs that help people with emotional problems. So visiting a psychiatrist may be necessary for this reason as well. (Check out the "Finding a Therapist" and "Treating Emotional Problems with Medication" sections later in this chapter for more information.)

Determining If Your Problem Is Anxiety

Your emotional problem may not be depression. You may be facing anxiety. *Anxiety* is an active feeling of dread, panic, and powerlessness, compounded with a sense of doom and overall foreboding. It's different from depression, which is a feeling of flatness and hopelessness. Because the symptoms of fibromyalgia can be so unpredictable, sometimes, FMS may create or enhance already existing feelings of anxiety.

Defining anxiety

Do you feel like you must do *something,* but you aren't sure *what?* Are you often in a state of panic? If so, you may suffer from an anxiety disorder.

Tina has fibromyalgia, and she's also suffered from frequent occurrences of her heart racing uncontrollably and feeling like she might faint. But the doctor said that her heart was fine. Tina consulted with a therapist who suggested *cognitive behavioral therapy,* a form of "talk therapy," in which people discover how to identify negative ways that they're reacting to life problems. With the help of her therapist, Tina learned to avoid panicking over minor problems. The therapist also helped Tina challenge her idea that illness is a deserved punishment, freeing her to actively work on resolving her fibromyalgia symptoms. She became more proactive about resolving her FMS by practicing relaxation therapy. (Read more about relaxation therapy in Chapter 13.)

Treating anxiety

You don't have to suffer from anxiety. Sometimes, medication, such as anti-anxiety drugs, can help with anxiety, and, sometimes, therapy can help. Many people find solace in talking to others with similar problems. (Read about support groups in Chapter 18.) Others find that one-on-one sessions with therapists work for them (see the "Finding a Therapist" section later in this chapter). The same coping method isn't effective for everyone, and the first one that you try may do nothing for you. The important thing is to continue to seek emotional health, and eventually, you'll find it.

Taking Your Emotional Temperature

Some people have said that when you're up to your neck in alligators, it's hard to remember that your original goal was to drain the swamp. Whether you know that your own "alligators" of problems are currently overwhelming you or you're not quite sure (or maybe you're completely oblivious!), my emotional temperature test lets you see how you're doing emotionally.

In the preceding sections, I talk about what depression and anxiety are, but now, you can take a look at some everyday examples of emotional distress. If any one of these situations describes your emotional state, you may be experiencing depression or anxiety.

✔ **Nearly every morning when I wake up, I feel like crying or screaming and going back to bed.** If you wake up feeling sad, you may be depressed. When you have fibromyalgia, the pain and insomnia may be what's gotten you down. Or you may have a combination of FMS symptoms *and* depression. Talk to your doctor about this.

✔ **My family and friends constantly ask me if I'm okay. I tell them that I am, but they seem unconvinced.** If your family and friends keep asking if you're okay, maybe they're noticing behavioral indicators of an emotional problem, such as you never smile and often (or always) seem extremely distressed. Pay attention. Maybe you're getting a "yellow light" warning signal that you should heed before you plunge into dangerous "red" territory. Talk to your doctor or therapist about this.

✔ **At least several times a week, I find myself wondering if my life is really worth living.** Everyone wonders once in awhile about their overall value to the cosmos. But if you find yourself constantly questioning your personal self-worth, you may be in, or headed for, a depressive state. If you've been thinking about suicide on top of these feelings, you need to talk to a doctor or therapist right away.

✔ **I feel like a robot. I get up, go to work, and come home. It's all so joyless.** If you see your life in shades of gray and feel like you're nearly always operating on "automatic pilot," this is an indicator of depression. It's a sign that you need a break. Try to change some patterns in your life. Call one or more friends and arrange to go out with them. If this idea has no appeal, you need to see a therapist.

✔ **I can't think of anything I'd like to do tomorrow or anytime in the future that makes me feel really excited and happy.** If nothing makes you happy, and even thinking about activities that you used to like gives you no reaction, you're either depressed or stressed. You could also be *both* depressed and stressed. You need to see a doctor or therapist.

✔ **A lot of times, I feel like if one more person aggravates me, I may explode.** Anger is one way that some people exhibit depression or anxiety. If minor slights get your blood pressure up or make you want to put your fist through a door, don't wait to see a therapist. Call now.

✔ **I've been eating a lot more than I used to eat (or a lot less), and my weight has changed considerably in the past few months.** Overeating or undereating can often be signs of depression or of emotional distress or anxiety. If you haven't tried to gain or lose weight, but it's happening anyway, see your doctor. If medical problems are ruled out, a therapist is often your next best choice.

✔ **If a magic genie offered me three wishes, I'd have trouble thinking up even two requests. Or maybe even one.** If you couldn't even think of one or two things you'd want if three magic wishes were offered to you, you may be depressed. Get a physical exam to rule out hypothyroidism or other medical problems. If your tests are normal, see a therapist.

Finding a Therapist

When looking for a therapist, you'll find many different therapists with different orientations. The key is to find a therapist who understands your particular problems, and who can help you create a plan to deal with them as effectively as possible.

One very important aspect of your therapist, no matter who you decide to work with, is that the therapist must realize that FMS is a real pain disorder. Your anxiety or depression may be exacerbating your pain and other symptoms of fibromyalgia. Conversely, your fibromyalgia may be worsening your emotional symptoms.

The pain is no figment of your imagination. If the therapist has experience working with patients with FMS, then fine. But you may also do well with a therapist who has an open mind and is willing to find out about fibromyalgia.

Suppose that you've found a good, credentialed therapist. Will she make your problems go away or turn you into a new person? A good therapist will help you identify your key problems and create an assault plan to tackle them. Therapists aren't superhuman, but they often know ways to help you manage your problems. Don't expect overnight results, which may be hard to accept in an era of email and faxes. But resolving emotional problems takes time.. How much time? It's impossible to say, but probably at least five to six sessions, at a minimum, and over a few weeks or a month.

Sorting out mental health professionals

Many people are confused by which professionals can provide help for emotional problems. There are four primary types of helping professionals, and they vary according to their educational background, the types of patients they treat, and whether they may prescribe medication. (Only medical doctors can order medicines.) They have other differences between them as well.

  ✔ **Psychiatrists:** Psychiatrists are medical doctors who treat emotional problems, and as such, psychiatrists are the only therapists discussed in this section who can prescribe medication. Some psychiatrists treat only children and adolescents or only (or mostly) people with specific types of problems. Most psychiatrists treat a broad range of emotional problems. Many psychiatrists don't spend a lot of time on "talk therapy," although some do. In general, appointments last a half-hour or less. A "medication check" for established patients may last a few minutes.

✔ **Psychologists:** These are individuals with PhDs or doctorates in psychology or counseling. They are usually called "doctor," as in Dr. Freud, even though they don't have medical degrees. Psychologists may specialize in treating specific types of problems, or they may be generalists. Psychologists use many different types of therapies; however, the most effective one appears to be *cognitive-behavioral therapy*. This is a form of therapy in which the therapist teaches patients to identify their irrational and self-defeating ideas, and shows them how to challenge these ill-serving premises.

✔ **Social workers:** Social workers have a master's degree in social work (and sometimes a doctorate). Social workers are oriented to problem solving. Rather than delving deeply into why a problem exists, social workers are generally more interested in finding practical ways to resolve problems. Social workers may be adept at analyzing family relationships and helping individuals get along better.

✔ **Other therapists:** Some therapists have master's degrees in psychology or counseling. You should also check whether any therapist you're considering working with has a professional license with the state licensing board. (Most state licensing boards are at a department of professional regulation in your state capital.)

Finding and screening therapists

Suppose that you don't even know any therapists or how to find one. So where do you start in finding a therapist?

✔ Ask your doctor if she can recommend a good therapist. And don't worry that the doctor will blab to the world that you need to see a shrink. Doctors must hold your information in confidence.

✔ You can also call the *state Mental Health Association office,* usually in your state capital, for a recommendation. To find the nearest office in the United States, go to: www.nmha.org/affiliates/directory/index.cfm.

✔ Your clergyperson may also be able to recommend a therapist.

After you've found a potential therapist, how do you decide whether he's the one who can help? Here's a good place to start: When you call a therapist on the phone or see him in his office, tell him that you have fibromyalgia. If he says that his therapy will rid you of your symptoms, find someone else. Conversely, if he says that he may be able to help you resolve your emotional problems, he may be the right one for you.

Whether your therapist is an MD, PhD, MSW, or has other degrees, verify that he or she is state-licensed to practice. Most therapists proudly post their credentials on their walls, including college degrees and professional licenses. Make sure that you see them.

Meeting with a therapist

The first time you meet with a psychiatrist, psychologist, or other therapist, make the following determinations:

- ✔ Do I feel comfortable with the therapist, and think maybe he or she can help me? (If not, find another therapist.)

- ✔ Does the therapist have any experience with pain patients? (It's best to ask the therapist during the session, because the information may not come out otherwise.)

- ✔ What type of therapy is performed? (Ask the therapist. Keep in mind that cognitive-behavioral therapy is proven to be effective.)

Treating Emotional Problems with Medication

TV character Ally McBeal agonized over taking Prozac and ended up flushing a bottle of pills down the unisex toilet. Maybe Ally was right, in her case. But in the real world, medications for emotional disorders can provide considerable relief. In some cases of people who are severely depressed or anxious, medications can save lives.

Just because medications for emotional problems are needed doesn't mean that they're free of side effects. Every medication you take, including Tylenol, has potential risks to consider. (Check out Chapter 10 for a list of common side effects associated with antidepressants and anti-anxiety medications.)

Taking psych meds

Most people with FMS who also have emotional disorders suffer from either depression or anxiety. Just telling yourself to forget about your problems or smile through your tears isn't usually effective, unless the problem is a minor or temporary bad mood. Antidepressant medications may help alleviate depression and anti-anxiety drugs may help squelch anxiety.

You may need one or more drugs to combat your emotional difficulties. Your doctor will probably start you out on a low dose of one drug, in order to be able to tell which drug is responsible if side effects occur. Check out Table 16-1 for a list of common prescription medications for depression and anxiety and their most common side effects.

Table 16-1	Common Medications for Depression and Anxiety		
Medication	*Generic Name*	*Prescribed For*	*Most Common Side Effects*
Prozac	Fluoxetine	Depression and anxiety	Loss of sexual desire
Zoloft	Sertraline	Depression	Loss of sexual desire
Valium	Diazepam	Anxiety	Sleepiness, physical dependence
Effexor	Venlafaxine	Depression	Nausea, increased blood pressure
Buspar	Buspirone	Anxiety	Dizziness
Paxil	Paroxetine	Depression and anxiety	Nausea, sleepiness
Xanax	Alprazolam	Anxiety	Drowsiness
Wellbutrin	Bupropion	Depression	Increased energy, poor sleep

Antidepressant medications often have benefits for people with fibromyalgia in addition to the emotional aspects:

✔ Depression increases the experience of pain, possibly due to a depletion of serotonin. Even if you're not depressed, antidepressants can improve your serotonin production, and thus, decrease your pain.

Nonpsychiatrist physicians often prescribe low doses of antidepressants to their patients with chronic pain. (For more information about this use of antidepressants, check out Chapter 10.) But if you have depression *and* chronic pain, you may need a therapeutic dose to help you deal with both problems.

✔ People with fibromyalgia often don't get enough restorative sleep. Antidepressants may help resolve this problem as well. (Be sure to read Chapter 14 on sleep problems and what to do about them.)

Combating the stigma of psych meds

Some people have a tendency to make extreme judgments about psychological medications. On the one hand, such medications are dangerous or even evil. At the other extreme, some people think that popping a Prozac will radically change their lives, instantly switching them from a sort of black-and-white environment to dazzling color, as in the Wizard of Oz.

What many medications for emotional problems do, when they work, is make you feel okay or normal. They should *not* make you feel euphoric or like you can conquer the world. In fact, you may not really notice that you're feeling normal, just as, when you have pain and it stops, you often don't think about your nonpain. Emotional pain can be like that, too. When it's gone, you don't think about it because you're too busy with your life. You look back on your week and say to yourself, "That was a pretty good week."

Some people conclude that if medications for emotional problems make a person with fibromyalgia feel better, the problem must have really been in their heads in the first place. But people with fibromyalgia don't create their own physical pain. It's there, and it's real. Depression, anxiety, stress, and other emotional problems have the potential to severely amplify the existing pain and other symptoms of fibromyalgia, making you feel much worse.

Conversely, when medications and/or therapy for emotional problems work, they can help to decrease your pain to where it would have been if you'd not been depressed or anxious. Sometimes, the medication may decrease your pain even further than that — but don't assume that all pain will disappear forever. Feeling better is what you should seek, not a total cure.

Part V
Living and Working with Fibromyalgia

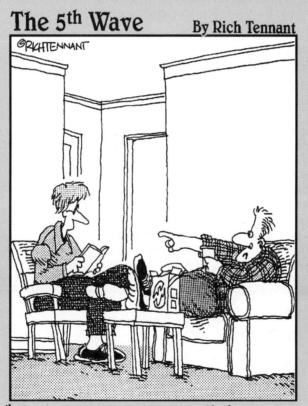

The 5th Wave   By Rich Tennant

"C'mon Darrell! Someone with fibromyalgia shouldn't be lying around all day. Whereas someone with no life, like myself, has a very good reason for doing so."

In this part . . .

Because fibromyalgia affects you pretty much 24/7, both on the job and at home, this part addresses both arenas of your life. In Chapter 17, I cover fibromyalgia on the job and what to do if your symptoms bother you so much that it's hard (or impossible) to work anymore. I also offer tactics on coping with your insurance company, your boss, your coworkers, and others.

Face it: Your fibromyalgia affects your family. In Chapter 18, I explain how your fibromyalgia affects your loved ones and what to do about it, including how to explain fibromyalgia to your children, what to do about your (possibly) impaired sex life, and other key issues. Chapter 19 is for non-fibromyalgia people: those who don't have the problem themselves but really want to help friends and family who do. I provide comments from people who have fibromyalgia on what they wish others would know, and I offer helpful hints on what to say (and *not* say) to a person with fibromyalgia. If you have fibromyalgia, you may want to discreetly leave the book open to this chapter for some key people in your life. I also include a chapter on fibromyalgia in children, and yes, they can and do suffer from this aggravating medical problem — yet so often, children and adolescents go undiagnosed. I hope Chapter 20 will help rectify that misperception.

Chapter 17

Working with Fibromyalgia — Or Going on Disability

*E*va hasn't told her boss about her fibromyalgia yet, and nobody else in the company knows about it so far, either. Eva's keeping her fibromyalgia a big secret, afraid that she won't be allowed to do her job if people at work know about her fibromyalgia. Eva often works alone, using a company-owned all-terrain vehicle to get to remote work sites where she does her field research. The vehicle has broken down a few times, and she's had to hike out of the wilderness to get help on more than one occasion. Eva's afraid that if the boss knew about her medical problems, he wouldn't allow her in the field alone — and Eva may be right.

Eva also performs extremely detailed work, and sometimes the *fibro fog* (difficulty concentrating) is so thick upon her that she has to double- and triple-check her work. So far, Eva's careful work has paid off, and she hasn't made any mistakes. But she fears that just the possibility that she may make mistakes is another reason to not tell anyone about her fibromyalgia.

Is Eva right or wrong about not telling her boss about her fibromyalgia? That's a tough call to make. She's doing her job well, and so far, nobody's even suspected that she has a problem. However, Eva worries about "what if" — so much so that her overall quality of life and general happiness is impaired. And if she ever *should* have a problem and try to make a claim, the company can say that Eva never told them about her fibromyalgia or her symptoms and problems.

Perhaps Eva's life would be a lot easier if she just came clean and told her boss about her problem with fibromyalgia. If she told her boss in a TV sitcom world, he'd understand completely, everyone would pat her on the back, unseen people would clap, and the camera would fade out. But life isn't always like that, and Eva knows it. So for now, Eva plans to continue to hide her fibromyalgia and deal with its symptoms as best she can.

As Eva's story makes clear, dealing with fibromyalgia in the workplace presents a unique set of challenges. In this chapter, I give you some guidance about how to handle work and fibromyalgia syndrome (FMS). I also give you some advice about what to do if your work burdens are so severe that you can't work full-time anymore and how to go about obtaining disability payments, if you need to take that step.

Explaining Fibromyalgia to Your Boss and Coworkers: Should You?

Telling your supervisor and coworkers why you're taking more sick days than anyone else and why you can't always perform at your peak level may seem to you (or to others giving you advice!) to be the obvious choice. But deciding whether to tell your supervisor and others at work about your fibromyalgia can be a dilemma. Will your coworkers think that you're an invalid or very disabled? Will they treat you differently? Or will telling them make your work life much better, and solve a lot of the problems that you're now facing?

In general, the reaction of people at work probably won't fall into the two extreme scenarios that you may envision. Telling your boss and coworkers about your fibromyalgia generally won't solve all your problems. And, on the other hand, it usually won't create cataclysmic new problems for you, either.

Karen says that she recently told her boss about her fibromyalgia. She's an editor, and, sometimes, her work schedule must be sharply reduced because of her FMS symptoms. For example, on many days, she can work no more than five hours per day, and she says that the pain and fatigue sometimes impair her concentration. Karen says that before she revealed her problem with FMS to people at work, she often came under intense pressure to work very long hours, but she just couldn't do it. Now, her problem with fibromyalgia is out in the open, and Karen can limit her hours.

Karen's boss accepts her plight, but her coworkers can't seem to fathom what fibromyalgia is and how it affects her — especially when they feel like they have to pick up the slack from the work that Karen's unable to do.

Maybe she's paranoid, but she feels like she's noticed that some conversations seem to stop when she walks into the room, and she's noticed a few resentful looks. Karen's thinking about talking to her coworkers more about her fibromyalgia, but she isn't quite sure what to say.

Deciding to tell/not tell

Here are some questions to ask yourself in deciding whether to tell or not tell your boss and/or your coworkers about your fibromyalgia:

- ✔ **Are your symptoms making your work quality suffer, so that people are wondering what's wrong?** If you can still handle the job and don't want people to know about your FMS, you can probably keep your secret. But if your work isn't quite as good as it once was, it may be best to explain why. Otherwise, people will supply their own reasons, and you may not like the reasons that they imagine are true.

- ✔ **Is the job itself worsening your symptoms?** If you work on an assembly line or have another type of job that makes your symptoms worse, you should think about your health. You can ask for a different job, shorter hours, or other changes when doing so for health reasons. Otherwise, things probably won't change.

- ✔ **Are you able to work as many hours as the job requires?** Sometimes, the fatigue and pain of FMS may drag you down. You may need to request other arrangements or even consider a different job in the company. (Or out of the company.)

Forming an explanation

If you decide that you want to talk about your fibromyalgia with your boss, and maybe your coworkers as well, what's a good explanation? I recommend that you say that you have fibromyalgia, which is a chronic, widespread pain problem that's accompanied by fatigue and, sometimes, other symptoms as well. Tell your boss that a doctor has diagnosed you with this illness, and you're frequently in pain, but you'll do your best to manage your workload. But also explain that, sometimes, the pain and fatigue may make it impossible for you to continue working, and you'll need breaks, or may need to stop working altogether. Sometimes, people will initially feel uneasy around you. But when they see you soldier on without a lot of self-pity and complaints, they may express a newfound respect for you.

Deciding Whether You Should Stay at Your Job

When you have FMS, you may sometimes feel like you're trying to press forward against a stiff wind, as you struggle to maintain a delicate balance between fulfilling your work commitments and coping with your fibromyalgia symptoms. Some people with fibromyalgia have been able to create an alternative work arrangement with their company to let them telecommute. Others have switched to flex time or to part-time work, and that option has enabled them to continue working in their jobs. Others, however, continue to struggle, afraid to tell anyone at work of their medical problem.

Alternative work arrangements can be great — if they're possible. But some jobs simply aren't adaptable to telecommuting, part-time work, or even *flex time* (when you set your own hours). For example, if you work with others on a team, the team members usually need to be there all at once. If you work in an office that needs to be staffed from 9 to 5, you can't work the night shift, although you may be able to work part-time during the day.

Working at home works for some FMS sufferers

Carla, a programmer, says that she would've had to go on disability if her company hadn't agreed to allow her to telecommute. She says that she couldn't handle the long commute anymore. She had almost nothing left, energy-wise, by the time she arrived at work, and getting home after a long day was a nightmare.

Telecommuting is a great option for many individuals who find commuting, and working away from home, to be difficult to impossible. But don't expect an ideal world if you work at home. Your coworkers may be resentful, for one thing. That's what happened to Jennifer, who says that she was put on salary, so that she could work at home rest when she needed to. Jennifer usually puts in more than the 40 hours she used to give the company when she worked in their building. But she says that her coworkers complained that it was "favoritism," and

they don't seem to understand that the change was made to benefit not only Jennifer, but also the company. Of course, Jennifer doesn't see her coworkers much because she goes into the office only briefly every week or every other week. She's decided that she won't worry about their jealousy.

Not all jobs are conducive to working at home, such as teaching (unless you're home schooling your own child), and many other careers. However, if at least some aspect of the job can be performed at home, as is often the case, people with fibromyalgia say that telecommuting can help a lot in keeping them continuously employed. They *do* still have to complete some amount of work within a given time, and they need to be people who are self-motivated and willing to push themselves when necessary.

Considering the Family and Medical Leave Act

The *Family and Medical Leave Act* (FMLA) is a federal law that directly affects workers in most companies. This law allows workers to take up to 12 weeks of *unpaid* time off each year for medical problems that they face or to provide care to members of their family. If you take an FMLA leave, your company must also hold your job open for you or give you a comparable job when you come back to work.

Such time off can be intermittent, meaning a day off here and there, and doesn't have to be weeks at a time. However, if you want to use FMLA provisions, you must inform your supervisor of your medical problem, and you should try to guesstimate how much time off you'll need. For further information on the Family and Medical Leave Act, contact the Equal Employment Opportunity Commission 1801 L Street NW, Washington, DC 20507; phone 202-663-4900; Web site: `www.dol.gov/esa/fmla.htm`.

Sometimes, the demands of the job may become impossible for a person with fibromyalgia. For example, Julie was a potter several years ago, but she had to quit pottery work. She explains that clay is extremely heavy, and she became exhausted after trying to work on the clay or even center the clay on the wheel. Often, she wouldn't go into her studio for days from sheer exhaustion. The gallery owner whom she sold her work to was angry because Julie's pottery was very popular, and the owner had actually wanted Julie to *increase* her production. But Julie just couldn't continue. It hurt too much.

So how do you know whether you have the kind of job that's usually not workable with fibromyalgia? Here are some questions to ask yourself:

- Can you take regular breaks at work, as needed?
- Can you be absent from work as needed?
- Do you need to move heavy objects or operate heavy machinery?
- Is your job especially sensitive to errors?
- Does your job require you to maintain painful body positions?
- Are others at work dependent on you being there regularly?

If you decide that you just can't stay on at your job, you have some new decisions to make. Can you work at another job in the same company? Or can you work part time? Maybe you'd be better off at another company. And if your symptoms make it difficult or impossible to continue to work, you need to consider applying for disability payments, covered later in this chapter.

Getting Your Insurance Company to Pay for Treatment

Most insurance companies know that fibromyalgia is a valid diagnosis and a real medical problem. But they may balk when you request medical coverage for treatments that they may see as "iffy," at best, or if you seek coverage for a screening test or a procedure that they don't generally cover. Because treatments or procedures that your doctor thinks you need may be difficult for you to pay for solely out of your own pocketbook, taking the time to convince the insurance company that your requests are reasonable may be worth the extra effort. This section offers advice on achieving that goal.

Providing more info

Sometimes, the initial claim for a treatment or test goes sailing right through your insurance claims department. But, sometimes, it gets flagged, and more information is required. The insurance company may send you (or your physician) a letter asking for more information. If more information is requested, the insurance company is usually specific about what they want. Often, you can call them and tell them over the phone what they need. Or you may be able to fax them the necessary information.

If you're able to fax information to the insurance company, always send the fax to a specific person. Insurance companies may be large and very busy, and losing things is very easy.

Understanding why your claim may be denied

The insurance company may deny your claim outright for an array of reasons. The company may decide that the type of claim isn't covered (such as for massage therapy or another type of service) because they've never covered it before. Or they may decide that the provider (doctor, chiropractor, or other person) isn't on their approved list, so they give your claim the old "denial" stamp. Or they may simply make a mistake and deny a claim that would normally be approved.

An appeal, however, will require another person at the insurance company to consider the treatment or doctor, and if you've backed your claim up, often you'll succeed. For example, if you can show that massage therapy or some other therapy may help, the person reviewing the appeal may give you the thumbs up. Maybe the doctor you want to see is the only person in the area who's knowledgeable about fibromyalgia, another reason to consider your claim. Offer facts that the average person may consider reasonable, and you have a better chance of successfully appealing the claim denial.

Appealing insurance denials: Do it!

The average person receiving a "denial" letter of his or her claim from the health insurance company is usually disappointed and takes no further action. If you think that the treatment you were denied was justified, don't make this mistake. Virtually every health insurance company has an appeals process, and appealing a denied claim with the hope that whoever reviews the appeal will reverse the decision is often well worth the effort.

The easy way

Sometimes, the mere act of calling the insurance company on the phone and simply telling them that you plan to appeal the denial may cause them to take a harder look at your request. Sometimes, you may be asked to wait, and then you may receive an approval that day or several days later. The reason: Few people like to have their work reviewed, and most hate having a decision overturned. When you appeal a denied claim, this automatically means that someone else, often a supervisor, will review their work, and could disagree with the initial decision. To avoid this possible outcome when you say you're going to appeal, the denying person may change his or her mind about your denial, transforming it into an approval. It doesn't always happen, but it's worth a try. If your denial stands, go ahead with the appeal.

If you talk to someone from your insurance company on the phone, always get the person's *name* and take notes. Write down the date and the gist of the conversation. Keeping this kind of a record can be very helpful later on, if Jack at the Hill Insurance Company says that no one's ever talked to you. You can tell Jack that you talked to Jill at the same company on May 25, and she said (whatever she said). Be confident and stand firm.

The hard way

Assuming that the verbal threat of an appeal isn't sufficient, you'll need to follow through. This may involve filling out forms that the insurance company provides. You should always include a cover letter that you write to go along with any required forms. In that letter, briefly explain what you want and why you think that you should get it.

In most cases, the notification that you received that denied your claim will tell you that you have the right to appeal, and will also tell you what steps to take. If that information isn't provided, ask the insurance company to send or fax you the form you need, or ask your HR department to help you locate the forms.

Don't expect instant results when you appeal a denial. It'll usually take weeks and may even take months before the case is resolved. Patience and persistence are your key allies toward succeeding.

Adding letters

Back up your appeal with information contained in a simple typewritten letter. Whenever possible, think of ways that the treatment you want (or the physician you want to see) would be cost-effective for the insurance company or even save them money. You may not care about that, but they do. For example, you may have been denied a referral to see a specialist, such as a rheumatologist or a neurologist. Or you may have been denied an opportunity to be evaluated with a screening tool, such as *magnetic resonance imaging* (MRI), or some other test that may help evaluate your condition. If you believe that seeing the specialist or having the test could better pinpoint your problem, and perhaps cut back on the number of physician visits you incur (and especially if it could cut back on costly emergency room visits), you should say so in your letter. If you can estimate the cost savings, do so.

Keep your letter to one page, if possible. Remember, it must be typewritten, not handwritten. If you can't type the letter because of an arthritic condition or another problem, get someone else to type it. Make sure that the letter is dated and that it includes your address, phone number, and employee health insurance number. Provide the name of your primary care doctor in the text of the letter.

Before sending the letter, carefully proof it to make sure that the letter has no spelling errors or typos. Nothing hurts a person's credibility like a poorly written letter that's full of errors.

Don't insult the insurance company in your letter, no matter how annoyed you may be with them. People, not computers, will read this letter, and they'll be much *less* likely to give you what you want if you call them fools, evil people, or use other forms of name calling (even if they deserve it).

Provide factual data. Tell the company what your diagnosis is and why you and your doctor think that you need the treatment, test, or to see the specialist who's not in your insurance company's network of doctors. State *exactly* what you want: Don't make the reader guess. You want coverage for an MRI or for a specific procedure or specialist. Also, tell them *why* you want it, even if the answer seems glaringly obvious. You want it because it can further determine what your problem is, it may provide pain relief, or whatever the reason. In addition, if such a treatment or referral was ever approved in the past, for you or anyone else you know with the same health coverage, say so. Provide as many details as possible. If the insurance company thinks that a precedent was set, they're more likely to give you what you want.

You may want to also ask your doctor to write a letter explaining why you need the treatment. Ask the physician to give you the letter, so you can refer to it in *your* letter. Provide the doctor's letter as an enclosure. If the doctor insists on sending the letter directly to the insurance company, ask for a copy. Refer to your doctor's letter in your letter, and enclose the copy.

If your doctor is in a clinic or office with many doctors, sometimes, one person there is responsible for pursuing insurance denials and approvals. He or she may be able to help you get approval for your claim.

Taking the Next Step If FMS Is Disabling

Perhaps you just can't continue on in your work because you're too sick or because the job requires more time and is more stressful than you can cope with — or maybe because of both reasons. If you're in bad financial straits and need money to support yourself, eventually, you'll have to apply for disability or take some other action to keep the dollars coming in. In that case, you may decide that the time's come to investigate a short-term or long-term disability leave from your job or to consider applying for disability payments received through the Social Security Administration.

A *short-term disability* can be an illness that prevents you from working anywhere from a few weeks to about six months, by most definitions. A *long-term disability* is generally a medical problem that prevents you from working indefinitely. However, corporate and state definitions of these terms vary.

When you have a disability, this means that a medical problem hinders or prevents your ability to work. You may need to file for a disability program, so that you can receive all or part of your income. You may also be too ill to return to work later on, and decide to apply for Social Security disability payments.

Disability programs fall into several major categories, and they vary in terms of how long they last, who administers these programs, whether or not the federal or your state government is involved, and in many other ways as well. These categories and their many rules and ramifications are far too complex for me to delve deeply into in one section of a book. But I can offer you a brief overview of disability options.

The skinny on worker's compensation

Worker's compensation (also known as "worker's comp") is for individuals who can't work because they were injured on the job. You may be eligible for worker's comp if you believe that your job contributed to causing your fibromyalgia — for example, if you have a job that requires repetitive motions. People with fibromyalgia are more likely to go with short-term or long-term disability options rather that worker's compensation, but it *is* still an option if you truly believe that your job caused your FMS. This program generally provides that employees receive about two-thirds of the amount of their paychecks. Nearly all companies have worker's compensation programs. Worker's compensation isn't a long-term option, however. Eventually, you must go back to work or apply for a short- or long-term disability benefit.

Questioning yourself

Each person must make his or her own decision about whether to apply for a disability. In general, don't think that your pain will automatically get better after you're on disability. Often, the loss of social function can have a negative impact on pain. Asking yourself the following questions as part of your decision-making process may help.

- ✔ Have you exhausted all possible therapeutic options that were given to you? Have you done everything you can to decrease your pain, including taking your medications, improving your sleep, and doing your exercises?

- ✔ Has your doctor told you that you should quit working or significantly reduce the number of hours that you work?

- ✔ Have you been taking more than four to five days off per month because of your illness?

- ✔ Are you staying the same or getting worse?

- ✔ If you're considering a short-term disability, will this time off enable you an opportunity to improve your condition?

Getting disability from work

You can often get short- and long-term disabilities from work. Not all companies have such programs, though. (But in general, medium and larger corporations are more likely to offer them as part of your benefits package.) If you receive a disability payment from work, you'll get part or all your salary. In general, if you're eligible for short-term disability, you'll receive your regular paycheck amount, which will be taxed. If you receive long-term disability, however, you'll receive a partial amount, but it'll generally be nontaxable. (Check with the IRS and ask for publication 907, "Tax Highlights for Persons with Disabilities," for clarification.)

Don't assume that you'd know if your company had you covered for disability. Ask your employer or employee benefits representative specifically about disability coverage.

Going on Social Security

The *Social Security disability program* is a lifelong disability program for those who can no longer work at all, and for whom the possibility of ever returning to work is very slender. This federal program provides a monthly payment, as well as Medicare, for those approved. You may qualify for a Social Security disability if you've worked enough in the past and have also paid into Social Security. In addition, other family members may also be eligible for benefits, such as your children under age 18 or your spouse who's caring for your child under age 16. Whether Social Security disability income is taxable or not depends on many different factors. Contact the IRS for further information.

You *will* need to document your disability. You know that you're really sick, and you're not trying to rip off your employer. But some people *are* fakers, and for this reason, proof of disability is required. You can't prove it on your own; instead, you need your doctors to back you up with written statements and other information the Social Security Administration requires.

It's especially important that you and your doctor document the ways your illness prevents you from functioning in your *occupation* — not just in a particular job. If pain prevents you from making pottery or responding appropriately to split-second decisions, and those are essential acts in your occupation (potter or police officer), write it down, tell your doctor, and make sure that the information's clear to your disability insurer or the Social Security Administration.

To find out more about Social Security disability benefits, contact the nearest Social Security Administration office or go to www.ssa.gov/disability. html. Another information source of "frequently asked questions," offered by the National Organization of Social Security Claimants' Representatives, is also available on this site.

If you're still able to work at least part-time, and your gross earnings are more than $780 a month in 2002, you automatically don't qualify for a Social Security disability. If you *are* approved for a Social Security disability, the average monthly payment as of December 2001 (according to the Chief Actuary of the Social Security Administration) for a person with one or more children was $1,360 plus Medicare benefits. Also, after you start receiving SSDI benefits, you can't collect worker's compensation or unemployment benefits.

According to the Social Security Administration, to apply for a disability, you need to provide the following information:

- ✔ A phone number where you can be reached as well as contact information for a friend or relative.

- ✔ A list of all illnesses, injuries, and conditions that make you unable to work as well as the date when you became unable to work.

- ✔ Names, addresses, and phone numbers for all physicians, hospitals, and clinics and the dates when you were seen. (Whether they were consulted for fibromyalgia or not.)

- ✔ A list of all prescription and nonprescription drugs that you take.

- ✔ A list of all the jobs you've had for the last 15 years, with a description of the job you were in for the longest period.

- ✔ A list of all the education and training you've received to date.

- ✔ Your complete medical records. (The Social Security Administration will request this from your doctor, or you can provide it to them.)

- ✔ Your most recent W-2 form, or, if you're self-employed, your most recent tax return.

- ✔ Information about family members applying for benefits, such as your minor children. (Their Social Security numbers and proof of birth dates are needed.)

Don't expect immediate action on your claim: A year or even longer may pass before any action is taken, and even then, no matter how strongly documented your application is, or how ill you are, you may be denied. The whole process has several layers of application/appeal, and experts say that it's very important to not give up too early. Instead, appeal to the *reconsideration* level, the next rung up the appeals process. When your claim is reconsidered, you may *still* be denied at this level — attorneys say that many people are. If you're denied again, don't be discouraged; just keep going. The next level up is when an administrative judge hears your case, and experts report that this point is where many people's claims prevail.

Of course, seeing the judge doesn't guarantee anything, and I can't promise you that you'll ultimately be granted a disability payment. But if you're denied at the application point and don't appeal, you'll never know what would have happened if you'd kept going. So stay the course.

The burden of proof

Because fibromyalgia isn't a listed impairment specifically defined by the *Code of Federal Regulations* (Appendix 1 of Subpart P of Part 404 of 20 CFR), if your claim is denied at a lower level and you appeal the denial, the Administrative Law judge must determine whether your condition meets or exceeds those conditions already listed, in terms of causing the same degree of functional limitations of a listed impairment. Under current law, the judge must give claimants increased credibility in assessing their own functional capacity. By properly documenting your claim, you stand an excellent chance for success, although the entire process may take as long as two years from start to finish.

Giving your docs a heads up is a good idea. Contact your doctors by phone or by letters to let them know ahead of time that you're applying for Social Security disability, so they won't be completely surprised when they're contacted by Social Security Administration officials asking for information about your medical status.

If you apply for a Social Security work disability and also file for worker's compensation or unemployment benefits while your claim is pending, this action may be considered by the administrative law judge as proof that, except for the work injury or unemployment, you remain fully employable. This may mean that you won't be approved for the disability.

According to Alec G. Sohmer, an attorney who assists individuals nationwide who have fibromyalgia and other medical conditions with obtaining SSDI benefits, the disability standard for adults is an *inability* to engage in any substantial gainful activity because of a medically determinable physical and/or mental impairment expected to last at least 12 months.

Finding an Attorney to Help You

Navigating the sometimes torturous path of applying for a disability from the Social Security Administration is generally not a path for the inexperienced or faint-hearted. Many people tell me that they needed the services of an experienced lawyer to guide them through the numerous dangers and pitfalls on the rocky way to approval of their disability claim.

Make sure that any attorney you think about consulting with is also an attorney experienced with disability claims: Don't hire someone who wants to learn on your time. Local support groups may be able to recommend talented attorneys who can assist you with your disability claim. You can also ask your physician if he can recommend a disability attorney who's experienced in helping people who seek approval for Social Security disabilities. Keep in mind that the attorney should be willing to work on *contingency*, meaning that she'll receive a percentage of the lump sum you'll receive if you are approved (back dated to an earlier date, to be determined by the Social Security Administration).

This means that, if approved, you'll receive a lump sum payment dated back to approximately when you first applied. Of course, your attorney, if you've hired one, will receive a chunk of that "change."

 If you decide to seek an attorney to help with your Social Security disability claim, make sure that the lawyer is a member of the *National Organization of Social Security Claimants Representatives* (NOSSCR). Contact NOSSCR at 6 Prospect Street, Midland Park, New Jersey 07432; phone 800-431-2804; Web site www.nosscr.org.

When you've found an attorney who appears to be experienced and knowledgeable about disability claims, you should still ask him or her a few screening questions before signing up. Here are some questions that you may consider asking your candidate:

✔ About how many people have you assisted with their applications for Social Security disability claims? (The lawyer should've assisted at least 20 to 30 people.)

✔ Of these, about what percent were approved by the Social Security Administration? (The percent should be at least a majority of cases.)

✔ About how many people with fibromyalgia have you assisted? (Because the numbers may not be high, don't count out the attorney if the answer is "zero." But award that attorney bonus points if he or she does have experience with helping people with FMS.)

Chapter 18

Helping Loved Ones Deal with Your Fibromyalgia

*L*iza says that her fibromyalgia is pretty hard on her family, in large part because they just never know what to expect from her on any given day. Will she have enough energy and a low enough pain level to go to the movies or on a picnic with them today? Or to attend the school play that her daughter has an important role in? Or is this going to be yet another bad day, when it's better to leave Liza alone in her misery? Her family doesn't know — but then, neither does Liza herself.

Gail says that on some days she can tackle tough problems at work and then go home and cook dinner that evening. Afterwards, on those good days, Gail's able to help her children with their homework. However, on other days, Gail can barely manage to raise her head from her pillow because the pain is so intense. Her children told her once that they see her as two different people: Healthy Mom and Sick Mom. They don't seem to like Sick Mom very much at all, although they struggle to be fair.

This chapter is about understanding and dealing with the effects of your fibromyalgia on people you live with and on others you care about. Of course, if a person has fibromyalgia, as some of your family or friends may, that person may be able to understand and identify with your problems very well. (Keep in mind the old saying "misery loves company," while not forgetting that fibromyalgia affects people differently, and one person's experience may be very different from another person's.) However, most people you care about probably *don't* have fibromyalgia, and they can only know what fibromyalgia syndrome (FMS) is like based on what you tell them.

In this chapter, I help you understand how to explain your problems with fibromyalgia to others you care about, whether they're your children, your partner, or other important individuals in your life. I also talk about expressing your needs to others and helping them understand how your fibromyalgia affects you. In addition, it's important for *you* to listen to your loved ones and hear how your fibromyalgia affects *them*. You may be able to make simple changes that can satisfy everyone. At the very least, you'll clear the air.

Understanding How Fibromyalgia Can Affect Your Relationships

Most people can grasp the basic symptoms of fibromyalgia, and they can also understand how fibromyalgia affects you, individually, in your daily life. Of course, people aren't solely rational beings; they have emotions, too. As a result, even if and when they fully grasp your problem logically, they may still have an emotional element to their thoughts about FMS that includes feelings of anger, resentment, sadness, confusion, and so on.

These emotions are normal in everyday interactions with family members who have problems. Even if people don't like these feelings or want to deny that they exist, the emotions are still there anyway. As a result, friends and loved ones who sometimes react negatively to the effects of your fibromyalgia on them aren't necessarily bad or stupid or mean — instead, they're just human. But you can help them to cope with your fibromyalgia better.

Here are some ways that your fibromyalgia may interfere with otherwise usually good interactions between you and your friends and family members:

- ✔ You may not listen to what they say (or even hear it at all) because listening is hard when you're in extreme pain. They may think that you're not listening because you're bored or because you don't care. You should tell them that you're having pain, and you simply *can't* listen well now. When you're feeling better, you'd be happy to listen to what they have to say.

- ✔ You may be more prone to saying *no* to doing fun things or managing your responsibilities when your fibromyalgia symptoms are bothering you a lot. But you'd probably say *yes* if you were feeling better. Explain your reasons for saying *no* to the people you care about, and also explain that you *want* to say *yes* and *would* say *yes* if you were feeling better.

✔ You may tend to agree to anything your family members ask for, if agreeing will make them go away and leave you alone. (For example, you agree to requests you'd normally say *no* to, such as a sleepover your daughter has asked to go to at the home of a friend whom you've never met and know nothing about.) Or maybe you'd agree if your 10-year-old son asked for permission to take the next space shuttle to Mars. Hey, why not! It'd be good for him, broaden his horizons. Fight this natural impulse to make things easy on yourself now because the long-term effects can be worse. Avoid making decisions when you're feeling bad. If you must decide, think about how you've decided on similar issues in the past.

Be honest with yourself and your family. Accidentally slipping into using your fibromyalgia to get out of obligations that you don't enjoy can be very easy to do. But if you turn down an activity and then find energy to do things that you like, your family will notice, and you'll undermine their sympathy. If you say *no* to going to the fast food restaurant with your family but on the same day, say "yes" to a friend who wants to lunch at a new gourmet place, that's an oops! Don't make that mistake.

Putting Yourself in the Right Frame of Mind

When people have chronic illnesses, such as fibromyalgia, they often hold one of two extreme and opposite thoughts, and either way, they perceive themselves as a victim and a person unlikely to move forward. First, some people may believe that no one in the world can possibly understand or appreciate what they're going through. Trying to explain the problem to other people isn't even worth the trouble because they can never understand.

The other extreme view that people have is that everyone *should* understand the problem and know how tough it is for them. People who adopt this viewpoint may become angry and resentful when others aren't as sympathetic as they supposedly should be.

Both extremes are unreasonable positions to take. For example, although people who don't have fibromyalgia really can't "feel your pain," they may have arthritis or another chronic pain problem and, thus, can understand what chronic pain feels like, even if it's not *your* chronic pain. On some level, they should be able to grasp your problem. On the other hand, people shouldn't be expected to automatically sympathize with poor you — even when those people are your own loving family members. You're setting yourself up for great disappointment if you take either of these polar positions.

To avoid taking one of these two extremes, think about how you generally regard other people in relation to your fibromyalgia. As people who are hopeless and who could never understand? Or do you lean more toward regarding them as hopeless people who *should* understand? Try to move toward the middle. Most people are trainable and can be educated on what fibromyalgia is in general and how it affects you specifically, as well as what you need them to do.

Opening Up for Some Honest Dialogue

Because fibromyalgia can often have an intense emotional impact on your family members and friends, you need to discuss with them not only the basic facts about what fibromyalgia is but also how it makes you feel. For example, having FMS may make you feel useless, angry, upset, and so forth. You also need to give the people whom you care about a chance to tell you how your fibromyalgia and its effects make *them* feel. They may tell you that they get frustrated, upset, and angry and that they experience a wide variety of other emotions as well.

Talking about feelings doesn't mean that the time's come to assess guilt or blame. This isn't "Judge Judy," and no one's on trial. In fact, it's best if you tell your family and friends that your illness is *not* their fault. Sure, they should already know that anyway, but sometimes, they need to hear it from you directly. In addition, you should also tell the people you care about that the symptoms of your fibromyalgia aren't *your* fault, either. (You may need to remind yourself of this fact, too.)

The key purpose of discussing your feelings about your illness — and listening to how your friends and family feel about your illness — is to understand and accommodate each other in the best way for all of you.

One way to uncover issues and problems so you can start working on them is to call a family meeting. You'll probably need more than one meeting; maybe one or two a week until family members seem to feel generally comfortable with the way things are. The meeting should include your partner, your children, and anyone else who lives with you. They may be reluctant or suspicious about this idea but, if you have to, insist on their attendance.

A family meeting, as with any meeting, should have at least a general topic. If you want to get people's feelings out in the open about your fibromyalgia, then tell them that's the subject you're going to discuss. Prepare yourself ahead of time to hear some negative comments — as well as some touchingly supportive ones.

The first time you have a family meeting, set some ground rules. Everyone is allowed to talk, even your 3-year-old. But no one is allowed to give a speech. Everyone should be polite, and no insulting or mean remarks are allowed. (A lot of information can be communicated without sarcasm, insults, and so forth.) No one's allowed to interrupt. Everyone can speak, but they need to give others a chance to talk. This rule will need to be repeated several times at first. After awhile, don't be surprised when you're admonished by your 8-year-old child if you interrupt or speechify! Accept the criticism in good grace.

Expect some hesitation when you start because, after all, people in your family may have bottled up or censored their feelings for a long time. You can start by asking each person, in a going-around-the-circle fashion, to tell you what bothers him or her the most about you're being sick. You can also ask each person what is the most important thing that he or she would like you to do when you're feeling well. You may be very surprised at the responses you get.

For example, the holidays may be coming up, and maybe you don't feel like going through the big ordeal of completely cleaning and decorating the house and preparing a big meal for all the relatives to come over and devour. But you don't want to spoil the holidays for your family. If you bring up your concern, you may find, to your surprise, that other family members say that they'd really prefer a holiday celebration for "just us." You could also ask everyone what one thing they most would like to do over the holidays, and it may be something easy, like driving around and looking at house decorations or going to a religious service. Satisfying your family doesn't always have to be hard.

Don't expect every family meeting to reveal amazing or even useful information. Sometimes, they won't. Also, sometimes, important dialogue may occur *after* the meeting when members interact with each other about how they never knew that the other one felt this way.

 Avoid trying to talk about your illness or resolve any difficult communication problems with your friends and family during those times when you feel really bad. Tell others that you're sick now, but you'll talk to them later on about these issues. And make sure you *do* talk to them later, as soon as you can.

Anticipating Difficulties

Sometimes, your children, partner, and others may react negatively or even very negatively to the effects of your fibromyalgia. They may also react negatively when you can't participate in various fun or work activities because you feel bad.

Some of the negative responses that people you love may exhibit are:

- **Anger.** Perhaps family members are mad at you, but more likely, they're angry at your condition because you can't do the things they want or need from you, such as things you used to be able to do.

- **Annoyance.** This response is a milder form of anger. It may occur because you can't go places or do things that family members want you to.

- **Frustration.** Family members get frustrated because they have to accomplish many tasks that you used to do, and they wonder when or if this problem is ever going to end.

- **Fear.** The thought that things may get even worse drives fear. Will you become even more dependent on them in the future? Will you ever get any better, or will you only get worse?

- **Resentment or suspicion.** Maybe you don't have to wash the dishes, do the laundry, take the dog out, or do any other boring jobs that are part of every household. Your friends and family can't see the pain, and may begin to wonder if it's really there.

You know how bad you feel, and you probably also know that your family members are frustrated and upset that you can't do activities with them that may have been easy for you to do in the past. You can't help being sick, and it's not your fault. But your partner and your children may find it hard to cope with the effects of your illness, especially if they don't understand why you're in pain. It's important for you to understand and accept this fact.

Knowing How to Respond to "Helpful" Comments

Denise says that she's tried to explain how her fibromyalgia makes her feel to her friends, but they often respond by telling her that she should eat a healthier diet or get herself into better physical shape. One friend said, "Oh, fibromyalgia. That's what doctors say when they want to tell you that you have something, but they don't know what." Denise says that these kinds of comments really hurt her.

So, what do you do when people say such things? You have two primary choices. You can say nothing and let it bother you inside. Or you can say something, preferably something that won't antagonize your friends but will clear the air. Table 18-1 has some suggestions for how to respond to comments that you'd rather not have heard to begin with.

Table 18-1	What People May Say to You, and How You Can Reply
They say . . .	*You can respond . . .*
You should eat a healthier diet.	Even the best diet in the world can't make fibromyalgia go away forever.
I've heard that fibromyalgia is fake.	I've heard that, too. But it's wrong. Fibromyalgia is a real medical problem. Studies have shown this.
If you lost weight, that would solve your problem.	Losing weight probably would make me feel better, although it wouldn't cure my fibromyalgia. And exercising can be very hard when you're in pain.
Mind over matter is what I always say! Think yourself well.	A positive mental attitude is a good thing. But it can't cure chronic illnesses like fibromyalgia, arthritis, diabetes, and others.
You should try _____. (Fill in the blank.) It will make you better.	Some remedies work well for some people, and they don't work at all for others. I'm following my doctor's recommendations.

Helping Your Significant Other Cope

Fibromyalgia is very tough on you, but it's usually no day at the beach for your partner, either. Often, you can't do your share of the housework, and you may not be able to work full-time, part-time, or at all anymore. If you have children, your partner may have to take them places and resolve their petty squabbles — as well as participate in the fun stuff, such as watching your child win a prize or make a touchdown, without you because you're too sick.

Fibromyalgia can also put a major crimp in your sex life. Who wants to make mad, passionate love when your body feels like you contracted the flu — right after you were run over by a truck? Probably not you. On the other hand, your partner still *does* feel like having sex sometimes. In addition, he or she also needs some personal attention, too. Your partner needs you to listen when he or she needs to discuss work and family problems, as well as fears, goals, and aspirations. But listening and interacting can be hard to do when your brain seems to be stuffed with cotton balls and you feel like the village idiot. (If you're really feeling out of it, tell your partner that you'll talk to him or her later. And then do it, as soon as possible.)

The key is to share your feelings, without blaming your partner or yourself for your medical problems, and to also *listen* to how your partner feels, without taking offense to what is said or feeling as though you must defend yourself. Using that tactic, Colleen says that her husband Tom told her one day that he felt very sad and left out because she saved up all her "smiley face" time for everyone else but him.

Colleen thought a lot about what Tom said, and she realized that he was right. She'd been expending all her energy on their children or her coworkers and job. By the time her husband came home at night, Colleen was nearly always collapsed on the sofa, virtually incapable of any communication and only good for staring blankly at the television set.

Colleen decided to cut out some of her activities. For example, she arranged for other parents to drive her daughter to soccer practice and her son to Cub Scouts. At work, when asked to collect money for charity, she said that she couldn't do it this year. Colleen also cut back on her work hours, deciding that her own health and her relationship with Tom were more important than trying to be a fast-track worker. Colleen also learned to say, "No, I can't do that." She discovered that, in most cases, she didn't need to apologize or give 47 reasons why she couldn't do something. She just had to politely refuse — that was enough. This was an amazing revelation to her.

Another change: Colleen resolved to *not* try so hard to hide her fatigue and pain from others. Like many other people with fibromyalgia, she hadn't ever mentioned her problem to others, so they'd assumed that she could carry a full load. Hiding her pain and fatigue had been exhausting. She stopped hiding it, and now they knew. After they found out about Colleen's fibromyalgia, the demanding expectations of her coworkers decreased. With these changes, Colleen managed to hold on to some of her energy for Tom when he came home at night. Things were a lot better between them after that.

And what about sex? As with many people with fibromyalgia, Colleen's sex drive was usually slim to none, although she hoped that her reduced schedule might eventually change that. She also decided that she didn't have to feel 100 percent like having sex to participate in it with Tom. After all, if she waited for intense passion to overwhelm her, they might *never* have sex. Colleen talked to Tom frankly about sex and her problems with fibromyalgia. She asked Tom to be very gentle and take it slow when they had sex, and he agreed. She was surprised to find out that, sometimes, even though she'd been feeling pretty blah about sex, her interest was aroused after they started. Of course, when Colleen's symptoms were really bad, sex just wasn't going to happen. And Tom understood and accepted that fact.

Explaining FMS to Your Kids

Debbie says that she wishes she could just be a normal mother — she'd like to go outside and play basketball with her children, for example. She feels that she's deprived her children of a lot of their childhood because they've had to take on extra chores that she just can't handle. She's also not so sure that they really understand why she feels so bad much of the time.

Sometimes, you have trouble understanding fibromyalgia yourself. You may feel terrible on some days, okay on others, and, once in awhile, almost normal. It doesn't seem to make sense. So how can you explain this seemingly nonsensical problem to your children? It's doable! Read on.

If you lose your temper, largely because your symptoms of fibromyalgia are making you feel so bad, and you blurt out mean words to your child, just apologize. Don't wallow in guilt, don't castigate yourself out loud as the worst parent on the planet, and don't spend a lot of time explaining or trying to excuse your behavior. Just say you're sorry. That's usually enough.

Keep it simple

Most children, including adolescents, don't need a lot of complicated and theoretical explanations about the causes of fibromyalgia, symptoms that people experience, and so forth. They don't need charts or diagrams, and you shouldn't expect them to read books on fibromyalgia, either. (Although if they *want* to read something about FMS, this book is a good start.)

Your children need to know that your fibromyalgia is a chronic medical condition, and they also need to know how it affects you personally, what your specific symptoms are, and what they can do (or shouldn't do) to help you cope with your illness.

For example, if loud music really bothers you when you're sick, tell that to your children. They can use headphones, or they can turn the music down. And don't forget to ask your children how you can help them cope with your illness. For example, would they prefer to spend time at a friend's house when you're feeling your worst, or can they think of other solutions that work for you both?

Stress that it's chronic

Explaining the *chronic* part of your illness is very important because most children, and even many adolescents, consider medical problems as here today, gone tomorrow. A leg is broken, it's set in a cast, it heals, and then it's fine. A person gets a cold, suffers from sneezing, coughing, and wheezing, and then he or she gets well. Unless a child suffers from a chronic medical problem herself, most children perceive illness as something that improves and then goes away. The fact that some illnesses do *not* go away, but instead, require continued treatment, can be a difficult concept for many children to master.

Part of the difficulty for children in understanding a chronic illness is their own time frame of reference, which is now and, perhaps, later. (And *later* means this afternoon or tomorrow. It usually doesn't mean weeks or months from now, and almost never means years from now.) This different time frame of reference doesn't mean that they *can't* understand. It just means that explaining about a chronic illness may take more effort.

Clarify that they didn't make you sick

Be sure to tell your children, if they're still young, that your fibromyalgia isn't their fault. Children frequently have *magical thinking*, which means that they think that if they have "bad" thoughts, bad consequences can happen to other people. For example, your small child may think that you're sick because she was mad at you one day and wished to herself that you'd be punished. Tell your children that having angry thoughts flash through their heads is normal, even though it doesn't seem so nice. But having those bad thoughts can't make other people sick.

Another concern is that your children may think that your illness is fatal. They won't necessarily tell you that they're worried you could have cancer or another illness that can kill you. Joanie, whose mom has fibromyalgia, developed a fear of going home after school. She'd begun to fear that one day, she'd come home and find her mother dead on the couch. After all, Mom was so sick all the time. When Teresa, her mother, realized what was going on, she reassured Joanie. Yes, she was sick. But no, she didn't have a terminal illness.

Anticipate questions

It's understandable and normal if your children have many questions about your fibromyalgia. When you open the topic up to questions, you may be surprised at the floodgate that's released. Sometimes, questions will come right away. Sometimes, questions will come tomorrow or a week from now.

Your children may ask how long you're going to have this condition (you don't know) and when you're going to get better (you're working on it, but again, you don't know the answer to this question, as much as you'd like to), as well as many other questions.

Your children may ask you if they're going to "get" fibromyalgia, too. Although fibromyalgia isn't a contagious disease, certain studies indicate that FMS "runs" in families. However, the only way to know if someone has fibromyalgia is for that person to see a doctor.

Vary your approach with the age of your child. For example, if the child is up to about 8 or 9 years of age, you may want to use the analogy of a glass, giving a concrete example of you when you're "spilling over" with pain and tiredness. Fill the glass up in the sink and let it spill over. The glass represents you on a bad day. Then, fill it up short of the brim. This is you when you have some extra energy to give your family. Older children won't need to see a demo: You can explain the spilling-over concept in words. On one of your bad days, you can tell your children, "It's a spilling-over day for me today. Sorry!"

Joining a Support Group

Support groups can provide you with valuable information, moral support, and a feeling that you aren't alone. At the same time, some support groups can be constraining. And sometimes, people who attend support groups say that some people in those groups complain nonstop and offer no solutions to their problems.

Don't go by what others, including your best friends, think about particular support groups. Instead, find out for yourself. Take a "test drive" of a support group before joining up by attending a meeting, observing what happens, and seeing whether you think that you'd feel comfortable as a member.

Some areas have support groups with meetings that are moderated by professionals, such as psychologists and social workers. These groups generally cost money, but the presence of a skilled leader can enhance the effectiveness of the group and decrease the experience that people are "just complaining." If you can't find a good free support group, consider trying a professionally moderated group (if you can find one nearby). Your insurance company may even cover the cost. Ask your doctor if she knows of such a group.

Pros and cons of support groups

Nearly every type of support group, no matter what type of members the group is supporting, has both pros and cons.

If you're eager to hear the latest opinions on fibromyalgia treatment, from a layperson point of view, people in support groups often are among the first to know what's hot, what's worked for them, and what failed miserably. They may also be knowledgeable about the most recent studies, journal articles, medications, alternative remedies, and any other info you'd like to know about FMS.

Support groups aren't for everyone. On the downside, support group members may have little or no medical expertise, and they may be unable to screen out the scams from the bona fide treatments for fibromyalgia. So always take the advice of nonphysicians with a grain — or maybe a pound — of salt.

Lydia says that she went to a local support group for people with fibromyalgia several times, but she always felt much worse afterwards. Carmen says that the members of her support group were all so physically ill and miserable and hopeless that she couldn't stand to be in the room with them. She much prefers an online support group, where she can exchange ideas with others who are also sick but really trying to get better. Deanna says that she gained a great deal from her support group meeting: She heard about a great doctor who treated FMS. She called him for an appointment, was treated, and feels much better.

Should you take others with you to meetings?

If you find a good support group where you feel comfortable discussing your symptoms of fibromyalgia and where other members offer helpful suggestions on how to feel better, this group is one to treasure. Because you like it so much, you may think that taking your children, your spouse, or others to a meeting would be a great idea. By going, they could understand what fibromyalgia is all about. Taking people who don't have fibromyalgia with you to a support group has many pros and cons. I cover a few major ones here.

The key advantage of taking a person who does *not* have fibromyalgia along with you to a support group is that your partner or family member can see with his or her own eyes that many other people have the same kinds of

Getting e-support

Online support groups can take two forms: *list-servs* (Internet special interest organizations in which you receive all messages by e-mail) or *newsgroups,* which are areas on the Internet where people can read and leave public messages.

The two newsgroups that concentrate on fibromyalgia are alt.med fibromyalgia (an extremely popular group), and alt.med. fibromyalgia.recovery.info (another very popular group). Contact your Internet service provider to find out how to access newsgroups. Reading messages on the newsgroups doesn't cost extra, nor do you pay membership fees. Your only expense will be what it costs to use the Internet.

Fibromyalgia Community has a listserv. To find out about this group, go to www.fmscommunity.org and click on the listserv information link. Other listservs for fibromyalgia are described at this site: members.aol.com/fibrocloud/central.htm.

The key advantage to these groups is the wealth of information that's provided, as well as discussions about feelings and issues related to

fibromyalgia. In addition, participants frequently provide Web links that you can click on to move to interesting Web sites or to journal or newspaper articles.

You can "lurk" (read online messages without revealing your presence) or place messages yourself. Keep in mind that anyone who uses the Internet, anywhere on the globe, will be able to read your postings, so don't get overly personal. It's also important to realize that some people who post messages online are trying to promote a particular product that they may have a financial interest in. So keep your thinking hat on and your skeptical brain in gear.

Internet groups that discuss fibromyalgia and provide information can be treasure troves. But keep in mind that they're nearly always dominated by people who aren't physicians and who have no medical training. Reading the postings, as well as asking questions and receiving responses, can be educational and helpful. But don't take medical advice from people who aren't physicians. Always consult your doctor first before starting or ending any over-the-counter or prescribed medications.

symptoms and problems that you have. You're not an anomaly. In fact, you may be a lot better off than some of the other members, in terms of energy levels and how you're coping. If so, your loved one can gain a whole new view of how fibromyalgia can impact a person's life (and how lucky you both are).

You may also be worse off than other members, and that can be useful information to your family member or partner as well. He or she may not have realized how difficult your symptoms were and how hard you've been struggling to cope with your illness.

Taking your partner or loved one with you to a support group meeting also has some disadvantages. He or she may be uncomfortable and unhappy and may also become upset about viewing the misery and pain of so many people. Some individuals who *do* have fibromyalgia say that seeing the pain of others has distressed them greatly, so it's fair to say that a person who *doesn't* have fibromyalgia may also become very upset.

If a meeting (or most meetings) becomes a gripe session about how awful the family members, spouses, and partners are, your loved one will likely find the discussion to be very distressing, especially if that loved one is doing the best that he or she can to be supportive and helpful. Being perceived as the "enemy," when you know you're really trying to help, can be very hard to handle.

Children and teenagers may become upset and distressed about the frank discussions that occur in support groups. And they really don't need to hear individuals talk about their sex lives (or lack thereof).

Before you even consider bringing your partner, your child, your teenager, or anyone else who you love to your support group, attend a few meetings. Make sure that it's a visitor-friendly, or at least visitor-neutral, environment and one your loved one may gain insight from. He or she won't benefit from a mentality that sees people without FMS as the bad guys. But he or she may gain from an environment where people are open to sharing information in a positive manner.

Chapter 19

Helping Someone You Care About Who's Hurting

Carly doesn't have fibromyalgia herself, but her best friend Shannon has been diagnosed with fibromyalgia syndrome (FMS). So many times, Carly has wanted to sympathize with Shannon and with the pain, fatigue, and other symptoms that she's obviously going through. But Carly is often afraid to say something because she might say the wrong thing. Is Carly right to be so worried about being "politically correct" around her friend Shannon — that she's basically tongue-tied, even when Shannon is clearly hurting?

The answer is *no*. And yet, it's also *yes. No* because feeling like you're avoiding a topic that looms so large in the life of your friend or loved one isn't good. But *yes,* with regard to holding back comments, because many times, people blurt out comments that they think sound kind or helpful, but that aren't taken that way. For example, saying, "I know just how you feel," when you don't have a clue how the person feels, can be upsetting to a person with fibromyalgia.

In this chapter, I talk about how you can understand how friends, family, and others feel when they have fibromyalgia, without actually having fibromyalgia yourself, and what you can do to help them. I also talk about expressing gentle affection for the pain that your loved one is going through. But don't worry! You need not adopt a permanent "hands off" policy. I explain how to handle the touching/nontouching aspect of your relationship.

I also cover *your* feelings in this chapter, and discuss whether or not you should tag along to an FMS support group meeting for people. Going to such a meeting when you don't have FMS yourself has pros and cons that I describe .

Understanding Without Feeling Their Pain

Frankly (and please trust me on this one), if you don't have fibromyalgia yourself, you really don't want to "feel the pain" of someone else who does have it. The fact that your friend or family member has to put up with it is bad enough. However, because you can't feel how your friend or family member feels, you can't fully understand what she's going through with her symptoms. Instead, you must rely upon your observations of her behavior, what she tells you, and what you can find out about fibromyalgia. (This book is a very good start!)

Knowing what to say, what not to say, and when to say nothing at all can be a challenge. Should you express concern for how bad your partner feels or show sympathy with a smile? I can't provide you with one right answer for every situation, but the following section offers ideas that may help.

Sympathizing without saying that you know how FMS feels (you don't)

How can you be truly sympathetic when you can't really experience how your friend or loved one feels? You can talk openly with your friend about her FMS, asking questions, making supportive comments, and listening attentively. Try to understand what she's going through as best you can. Attempt to relate her problem with difficulties you've had, but other people didn't understand or relate to.

You'll never say the perfect thing at all times: No one does. But you can try to avoid saying annoying things, and work on making supportive statements.

Here are a few examples of what you can say to help a person you care about who *does* have FMS. (Use your own wording, of course.) These simple comments may help or, at least, may start a dialogue between you and your loved one. (See the sidebar entitled, "Helpful/nonhelpful statements to make to someone with FMS" later in this chapter for more helpful statements.)

> ✔ Fibromyalgia sounds really difficult to deal with.
>
> ✔ How can I help?
>
> ✔ I'm sorry that you have this problem.
>
> ✔ It must be hard to look normal, but feel really bad on the inside.

After your friend responds, summarize what she's said to you. Doing so shows that you've been listening. When you summarize what you think that your friend has said, even if you get it all wrong, at least the person can tell that you're making a sincere effort to understand and to help. For example, you may say, "It sounds like you're having a really hard time right now." Or, "This medical problem is not one for the faint hearted!" She may agree and try to explain her problem, or may nod in relief that someone cares.

Knowing what NOT to say

Avoid making comments that deny or diminish the pain of the person with FMS, such as "It can't be that bad!" or "Tomorrow will be a better day," and so forth. He or she feels really bad right now and doesn't need to hear comments that are unsupportive and hurtful. Read on for more information on what not to say.

For starters, do *not* say that God or fate or karma gives problems only to people who can handle them. Even if you think it's true, consider how negative such a comment may sound to other people. It sounds like you're saying, "If you're strong, you deserve to be punished for being strong."

Also, when talking with your loved one who has fibromyalgia, don't fall into an unconscious one-upmanship, or a "I know someone sicker than *you* are." (Say it in a sing-songy voice, like a child, to see how irritating it can be.) You may think that you'd never do this, but it's so easy to do! For example, if your friend talks about her pain and fatigue, don't say that, yes, that's pretty bad, but your sister's cousin's husband in Latvia *really* has a problem, because blah, blah, blah. Think how you'd feel if someone did this to you. If you start to say something that fits this bill, stop right away.

To better relate to your family member or friend who has fibromyalgia, remember how you've felt when friends or others have glossed over a distressing illness or another disturbing problem that you had. Maybe other people told you to cheer up and get over it or that it was really no big deal. Maybe you felt like you didn't have permission to feel the emotions you were experiencing or that they were wrong in some way. Re-experience the emotions you felt when your pain and loss was denigrated. And then work on *not* diminishing the feelings of your loved one with fibromyalgia.

Helpful/nonhelpful statements to make to someone with FMS

I can't cover every possible situation that may occur between you and your friend or loved one who has fibromyalgia, nor can I write you a script for the exact perfect things that you should say to your friend or family member who's hurting so badly. But I can give you some ideas of unhelpful comments to avoid and the helpful comments to make instead.

✔ **Nonhelpful:** I know *just* how it feels having fibromyalgia because I have _____ (Fill in the blank).

Helpful: I don't have fibromyalgia myself, but it sounds awful.

✔ **Nonhelpful:** If you exercised more, you'd feel better. You're out of shape.

Helpful: It must be hard to exercise when you're hurting. Maybe when you feel well enough, we could exercise together.

✔ **Nonhelpful:** Cheer up! Other people have it worse than you do.

Helpful: It's hard to be cheery when you're in pain. You don't have to put on a fake happy face for me.

✔ **Nonhelpful:** Maybe you need to go into therapy — right away.

Helpful: Sometimes, therapists can help with feelings that come with a painful chronic disease.

✔ **Nonhelpful:** You're only given burdens to suffer that you can bear.

Helpful: It's hard to know why people suffer difficult problems like the one you're having right now.

Leaving them alone: Sometimes, solitude helps

Sometimes, having company is great. And other times, it's not so great, like when you feel sick, cranky, overtired, and so forth. Normally, your loved one would love to spend time with you. But when her FMS symptoms flare up, sometimes, company is just too much to bear right then.

Lorna has fibromyalgia, and she wishes people would understand that she doesn't want them to try to "fix" her (she knows that they can't). Instead, she wishes they'd just leave her alone when she has a flare-up of her FMS symptoms. Lorna says that she does so much better by going into "hibernation" for those few days when her symptoms are really acting up. Afterwards, she can emerge and be much more congenial with her family and friends.

So how do you know when to steer clear of your friend or family member? Usually, it's not that hard to tell, when you know somebody. But here are some indicators:

✔ Your friend doesn't make eye contact. She could be angry or upset with you. Or she could be exhausted or in pain. Or all the above.

✔ His slumped over posture and dejected appearance connotes possible depression. But he says that he's "just tired," and may mean it.

✔ Your family member is responding in one-word answers and doesn't seem to be "here." She may wish to be alone

✔ Your loved one asks you the same questions repeatedly. She may be deep in a *fibro fog* (a temporary poor concentration, and a symptom of FMS) and may need some down time alone at home.

Avoiding too much contact: Even hugging can hurt

What's the normal and natural response when you're feeling sad for someone you care about who's in pain? For many people, their first reaction is to reach out to hug the hurting person.

Force yourself to resist the impulse to hug a person in the throes of a fibromyalgia flare-up. Even a little hug can feel like the grip of a grizzly bear to a person in pain from fibromyalgia. Always ask a person with fibromyalgia *first* if it's okay to give a hug. And if it *is* okay, keep it gentle. No bear hugs allowed, unless the person says that she wants one.

Just because you can't offer a person you really care about a big, enthusiastic hug doesn't mean that it's hands off forever. Instead, when your loved one is really hurting, a gentle butterfly-like touch to the shoulder or (preferably) hand can be seen and appreciated as the warm and affectionate gesture that you mean it to be. When your friend or loved one feels well enough, he or she will usually welcome a gentle hug. (But ask for permission first!)

Positive emotion and support can be communicated with other types of body language, such as:

✔ **Looking directly at the person as she speaks.** Most people don't look at each other because they're actually thinking of something else, like what they're going to eat for lunch or whether they should get those new shoes they saw in the store window. Try to really pay attention. People feel like you're really paying attention and you care about what they're saying when you look at them.

✔ **Smiling sympathetically, without making any comments.** This simple act shows your partner or friend that you're supportive and really care. A simple smile can mean a lot.

What people with FMS say they wish others would know, say, or do

Because you don't have fibromyalgia yourself, knowing what to say or do to help your friends or loved ones with aggravating medical condition can often be hard. Here's some advice from some people with FMS who've said (often quite fervently) what they really wish that others would know, say, or do.

Grace says that she wants people to know that she's really doing the best that she can, and on some days, just getting out of bed is a major accomplishment.

Charles says that he can't abide "whining" himself, but he thinks that it certainly helps if others can see that simple tasks require much more effort and discipline from a person with fibromyalgia.

Lola says that she'd like people to know that she really is in pain and isn't lying or faking it. She'd also like it if people wouldn't get upset if she forgets things or asks the same question ten times when she's in the middle of a fibro fog.

Frank says that it's important for other people to understand that their pain and exhaustion from other problems isn't the same as his. And also, just because he's feeling pretty good one day doesn't mean that he'll feel okay the next day.

Colleen says that she's already had her "head" treated. (She's seen a therapist for depression.) She'd like people to know that fibromyalgia isn't all in her head, but rather, it's all over her body.

✔ **Leaning forward slightly.** When people are really paying attention to what's being said, they often lean slightly forward and toward the person who's talking. This gesture will show your partner or friend that you're truly interested.

When you're talking to someone, you have your own basic "self-talk" going on in your mind. Whether your basic thoughts are trivial or very deep ones, you do your friend or loved one credit by actually listening to what she's saying and then responding. And if you can't listen now, because you're too stressed out or worried or tired or whatever, tell your friend that you're distracted now, but you'll really listen later on today or tomorrow or another specific date. And be sure that you follow through, too!

Pay attention to body language

Although words do matter, what someone says isn't the only thing that counts.

In addition to paying attention to what your friend or family member with FMS says, also pay attention to what she *doesn't* say: Watch her body language. These are gestures and postures that indicate how the person really feels, despite what she may say. For example, a person who's standing with her arms crossed over her chest is often annoyed or impatient. (Or both.) A person who's leaning forward toward you as you talk is truly interested in what you're saying.

Observe your loved one's body language when you're interacting with each other. For example, if you've asked her to go shopping or you've invited her to come with you to a family party, and she's said that she'd love to come, but you see that she's slumped over and her eyes are basically glazed over, here's the reality. The mouth is saying yes, but her entire aura is emphatically saying, "No!" Make some excuse about *not* going, and you'll usually see at least a glimmer of relief wash over your pal.

Coping with Your Own Emotions

You know that your friend, partner, or family member (or someone else you care about) is hurting, and you feel sad for them. You probably also feel some other emotions as well — some that you might rather ignore because maybe you don't feel so proud of them. I'm talking about negative emotions, such as anger, frustration, resentment, and so forth. Or maybe you feel guilty for being healthy when your friend or loved one is feeling terrible.

When you live with a person with FMS

When you're the partner of a person with fibromyalgia, being sympathetic, kind, and loving all the time can be hard. Here are a few guidelines for partners:

✔ If you find yourself occasionally flaring up or saying something that's mean or unfair, give yourself a "timeout" away from the person with FMS. Later, when you've cooled down, apologize.

✔ Try to help your partner work toward solutions to resolve his or her symptoms, but realize that it's not up to you to make everything better. In fact, you can't. You can offer sympathy and support, but when it comes to acting, the ball is in his/her court. Not yours.

✔ Ask your partner what he or she needs when they feel ill. Sometimes, others think that everyone somehow "knows" (or should know) what they need, whether it's a kind word or driving them somewhere because they don't feel well enough to drive. Or something else. You're not a mind reader, and this isn't a game. If you ask but your partner won't tell you what's needed, don't worry about it.

✔ Don't expect your partner to be superhuman. Often, you'll see him or her struggling with goals, and you may feel like the problem is that they're not taking good care of themselves. Although FMS patients greatly benefit from a disciplined lifestyle (exercising, eating right, sleeping enough, avoiding stress, and so forth), they can't possibly be perfect at all times.

Negative emotions are normal in life, and coping with them by confronting them head-on is ideal. Don't pretend that everything is perfect, and you really don't have these feelings at all. Instead, deal with the anger, frustration, and guilt so that you can better support your friend or loved one who's suffering. Read on for advice on how to do just that.

Dealing with anger

Anger is a common emotion for people who see those whom they care about in the grip of pain. Sometimes, you may get angry at the *person* who has fibromyalgia, possibly for complaining so much, and for seeming so totally focused on the pain — so that not much else seems to matter. Other times, you may be angry at the medical problem or the unfairness of it.

The best way to deal with your anger and to avoid a nonhelpful escalation of anger is to first acknowledge and accept that the fibromyalgia is here, and it's real. Next, try to pinpoint who or what you're really angry at. Are you angry with yourself for not being as understanding and caring as you think that you're supposed to be? Or are you angry at the person with FMS, for shutting you out and focusing on the pain and other symptoms?

After you determine who or what you're angry at, stand back and think objectively about what's going on. For some people, making a list of reasons why you're angry helps. (If you don't like the idea of making a list at all, then when you're alone, just state the reasons aloud.) Lists are easier to use, however, because you can forget what you've said later on.) Making a list may sound silly, but I recommend that you try this simple tactic anyway because you may find that it helps take some of the steam out of your anger and also clarifies what the issues are.

Write down, "I am angry because," and then just write down whatever comes to mind, without censoring your thoughts. You may find that you're angry because your friend or family member can't go to as many places with you as in the past or isn't as attentive as she once was to you and your own problems. Or the source of your anger may be something else altogether. Sometimes, you may think that you're very angry and upset about your friend and her sufferings with fibromyalgia, but the feelings actually stem from something that has nothing to do with her at all.

As you write, you may also find that you're not just angry, but you're also feeling sad, frustrated, anxious, and a host of other emotions. Identify and acknowledge these emotions. No, they won't evaporate, but they're often much easier to deal with when you realize how you really feel.

Fighting frustration

Feeling powerless and confused when you care about someone who has fibromyalgia is normal. These emotions fall under the category of *frustration*. Certainly, when someone you care about is in pain, excessively fatigued, suffering from a lack of sleep, and has many or all the other symptoms that are the features of FMS, you want to help. And when you can't think *how* to help, you're frustrated because you feel like you can't do anything.

You may wish that you had a magic wand that you could wave about dramatically, complete with magic words that you could also say that would instantly end all the torment for your loved one. Sadly, you and I live in the real world, and magic wands or special incantations won't make someone's fibromyalgia disappear.

 Positive thoughts and even prayer may help you deal with your frustration because they help you focus on your inability to magically resolve your loved one's problem and allow you to give up the illusion of control. The positive energy that's conveyed through prayer (or meditation) may also be helpful as well. If you're a religious person, you'll be comforted that your request to God will be heard. The problem will pass from you to God.

Getting rid of your guilt

Many people feel guilty when their friends, family members, or other loved ones are sick. They may have an irrational fear that they somehow *made* the person ill, through something that they did or didn't do and should have done.

Many people also experience a minor form of "survivor's guilt." If you're feeling pretty healthy and fit but your loved one is suffering a lot, maybe you wonder why you're fortunate enough to not be sick when your loved one, who's just as good of a person as you are, is suffering. Is it fair? No. But then illness isn't really a question of fairness at all.

You need to get rid of your guilt because it's not helpful for you or your loved one. It's not your fault that he or she's sick — you didn't make it happen. And it isn't your friend or loved one's fault, either. Even if you think that you were mean or uncaring at one point or failed to do something, that still didn't make your loved one develop fibromyalgia. Stress can make fibromyalgia symptoms worse, but it doesn't create this medical problem in the first place.

Get rid of your guilt by trying the following tactics:

✔ Adopting as a mantra the statement, "It's not my fault." (FMS in someone else really *isn't* your fault! Tell that to yourself and believe it!)

✔ Don't accept responsibility for alleviating your partner or friend's illness. You can provide sympathy and help. You can't cure him or her.

✔ Acknowledge to yourself what you *are* doing to help your loved one. When guilt feelings crowd in, think about how you drive her to the doctor's office when she's sick, cook dinner if she's too tired, and so forth. Give yourself some mental pats on the back. You deserve it!

Going to Support Meetings

Maybe your family member or loved one has suggested that you should attend a meeting for people with fibromyalgia, so that you can gain a deeper understanding of what it's really like. Or maybe you've come to this conclusion yourself because you want to have a better grasp of the problem and how your loved one feels. Maybe you can discover some new positive ideas that will help you to help your loved one feel much better.

Is attending a support group meeting for FMS when you don't have it a good idea? It depends. Ask yourself the following questions before you go to a support meeting with your hurting friend:

✔ Do you really *want* to go? If you do, fine. If you're just going because you feel like you *have* to go, and you'd rather watch grass grow or clean the attic (or some other activity that's not in your top 100 favorite things to do), think again about accompanying the person with FMS to the meeting. Sometimes, resentment can crowd out any positive feelings that you may have.

✔ Is it convenient to go, or are you making a heroic effort that may ultimately cause you some major resentment if you don't have a perfectly good time? If you think that you're making a giant sacrifice to go, think again about attending.

✔ Are you very curious about fibromyalgia and eager to meet other people with FMS, so you can better help your loved one? This mindset is a thumbs-up indicator for going.

✔ Can you cope with people in the group who may see you as someone who can't possibly understand or even as someone who's part of the problem? That can be painful to experience when you're trying so hard to help. Find out if other people who don't have FMS also go to meetings and if others (people who don't have fibromyalgia) are perceived as outsiders and intruders.

Chapter 20

Parenting a Child with Fibromyalgia

*T*ommy is an 11-year-old boy who's been diagnosed with fibromyalgia. He says that he's had aches and pains since he can remember, and he first found out that he might have fibromyalgia when his allergist noticed some possible symptoms and recommended that Tommy see a rheumatologist. The rheumatologist examined Tommy, ran some tests, and diagnosed him with fibromyalgia syndrome (FMS).

Tommy says that having fibromyalgia can be pretty tough sometimes. The pain and fatigue are difficult to put up with, and the other kids don't understand. His teachers haven't been very sympathetic either, and he thinks that most of them have never heard the word "fibromyalgia," or at least, not in relation to children. Sometimes, they seem to think that he's trying to get out of things, like homework assignments.

His parents *are* understanding, and that helps a lot, but he knows that they also worry about what's going to happen in the future, and whether he'll ever get better. He wonders about that himself, sometimes.

As Tommy's story shows, children can have fibromyalgia, too, although the juvenile version appears to have some differences from the adult kind, based on the few studies performed on children. In fact, in the case of children, their illness is technically called *juvenile primary fibromyalgia syndrome*.

In this chapter, I talk about what fibromyalgia is like in children, and I offer advice on how to help your child. I also talk about dealing with your other children who don't have fibromyalgia and avoiding the problem of them concluding that you have to be sick to get any attention around here. Communicating with teachers is another problem, as far as what to tell and not tell them to achieve the best outcome. Peers and what they think can also be a very tough problem, so, in this chapter, I also discuss ways to handle other children.

Keep in mind that, no matter how hard you try and how excellent of a parenting job you perform, you can't magically make the fibromyalgia go away, nor can you make everything "all better" for your child. Also (and this is important, so make it your mantra if you need to), it's not your fault. Help your child as much as you can, but realize that you can't make the illness go away.

Looking at Fibromyalgia Symptoms in Children

If you think that your child or adolescent may have fibromyalgia, what sort of symptoms should you be watching out for, and how is juvenile FMS different from or the same as adult fibromyalgia? In many cases, fibromyalgia in children is pretty much the same as FMS in adults. But pediatricians may dismiss muscle aches and pains and tiredness, saying that children are experiencing "growing pains," or they may ignore other symptoms, such as trouble getting to sleep.

In this section, I talk about the major symptoms seen in children with fibromyalgia, including some that are similar to and some that are different from, adults with FMS.

Showing fewer tender points than adults

Although the tender points of fibromyalgia (described in Chapter 8) are present when kids have FMS, some pediatric rheumatologists say that children with fibromyalgia have fewer tender points than adults, and the tender points that they do have are most likely to be found in the neck area. Children are less likely than adults to have tender areas in the lower back area.

Suffering from more stomachaches than adults

Some research indicates that children with fibromyalgia suffer from a greater incidence of stomachaches and abdominal pains than adults who have FMS. Perhaps the stress of fibromyalgia increases the rate of this problem, or maybe it's something else altogether. If your child is having many stomachaches, make sure that he or she gets a medical checkup.

Having poor sleep (like adults)

Most adults with FMS have a tough time with insomnia, and unfortunately, children with fibromyalgia share this symptom. Children with juvenile fibromyalgia may be more likely to have serious sleep disorders than other children. In a study of children diagnosed with juvenile fibromyalgia (reported in a 2000 issue of *Pediatrics*), researchers performed sleep studies of 16 children with fibromyalgia and compared their results to 16 children without fibromyalgia. The children with fibromyalgia had significantly more sleep problems.

For example, the FMS children took much longer to fall asleep, and these children had increased levels of wakefulness during sleep. Of the 16 children diagnosed with fibromyalgia, 6 were also positive for a sleep disorder known as *periodic limb movements in sleep* (PLMS). PLMS refers to an excessive level of leg movements while asleep. The researchers recommended that children who are diagnosed with juvenile fibromyalgia should be evaluated in sleep clinics to determine if they experience sleep problems that can be corrected.

In addition, it seems logical that children who are diagnosed with sleep problems should also be evaluated for possibly having fibromyalgia.

Is it FMS, or is it a way for a child to get out of going to school? One possible screening mechanism is to look for a sustained pattern of the symptoms of fibromyalgia experienced by most children. For example, if Susie or Jimmy Junior has aches and pains today, on a school day, but feels fine at the end of the day or on weekends and holidays, fibromyalgia most likely isn't the problem!

Discovering other key FMS symptoms

Experts say that if your child has all or most of the following symptoms, the underlying problem may be fibromyalgia. And these symptoms may be troubling enough that the child really can't cope with going to school on some days and with some children, on many days:

- Widespread pain
- Back and neck pain
- Joint pain without apparent swelling
- Fatigue
- Morning stiffness
- Frequent headaches
- Abdominal complaints, such as diarrhea or constipation

Accurately Diagnosing the Problem

Of all the groups of people who may have FMS (women of different ages, men, and children), children may have the most difficult time getting a proper diagnosis. This can make it hard on both parents and their hurting children. Diagnosing fibromyalgia in children can be problematic because

- Few people, including doctors, realize how prevalent it is. But about 2 to 8 percent of school children qualify for the diagnosis of fibromyalgia.

- Many pediatricians know little about the disease, and also, some don't believe that FMS is even a valid medical problem among children. It always must be something else, in their views. And if it's not medical, it must be a psychological problem. (Actually FMS *can* lead to depression, although that makes the fibromyalgia itself no less real.)

- Parents are unfamiliar with the diagnosis and, thus, they may find it hard or impossible to believe their children could have FMS. They may believe what others tell them — that FMS is just another fad diagnosis, the newest "flavor of the week" trendy disease. They're wrong but, sadly, perceptions can be very powerful. This means that children who do have fibromyalgia will continue to hurt.

The pediatrician or other physician should never rush into a diagnosis of juvenile fibromyalgia because your child may have another serious medical problem, such as arthritis, thyroid disease, an infection, an injury, or another medical condition. Doctors should perform a complete physical examination, take a complete medical history, and rule out other diseases with medical tests, such as tests of the blood or urine. Sometimes, the child will need more specialized tests.

After your child has been diagnosed with FMS, the next step is to find help for your child.

Getting Help for Your Child with Fibromyalgia

Suppose that you're convinced that your child has fibromyalgia. What do you do first? When deciding where to get help for your child, the best place to start is with your child's pediatrician, even though some pediatricians are wary of diagnosing fibromyalgia in children. If you find that your child's pediatrician is completely unsympathetic and unwilling to seek out the cause of your child's symptoms, you may want to identify another pediatrician. My guidelines for finding a new doctor, in Chapter 7, can be adapted to finding a new pediatrician.

Your child's pediatrician may also decide that the child needs to see another physician. In most cases, the child with the FMS-like symptoms should see a *pediatric rheumatologist* (or a pediatric neurologist), a specialist who's very experienced with treating joint and muscle disorders in children, including fibromyalgia. If your child needs to see a pediatric rheumatologist, your pediatrician can provide a referral for that.

A *pediatric rheumatologist* is a physician trained in medical problems of the joints and soft tissues and who specializes in treating children and adolescents with these problems. Arthritis and fibromyalgia are two conditions that pediatric rheumatologists treat.

Treating a Child with Fibromyalgia

Children with fibromyalgia are treated in much the same way as adults, although, of course, any medication dosages must be adjusted for children's weight, and the doctor should also take into account any other drugs the child is taking. When thinking about what medications to prescribe or what over-the-counter drugs to recommend to parents, doctors should always consider any potential problems that may occur to a person who's still growing and maturing. If the doctor doesn't mention it, ask her about potential side effects that can affect children. Drugs do have side effects, so no one should be nonchalant about prescribing medication for children.

It can be very hard on parents when their children have medical problems that others may be suspicious about. The child says that she's in pain or is too tired to get up, but your mother says that she's just lazy, and your uncle says that you're "coddling" her. Maybe you have some underlying doubts yourself about whether your daughter is faking it, and that she could be a hypochondriac. These attitudes are the same kind that adults with FMS have to face. But if the doctor has confirmed that fibromyalgia is present, assume that it's real. And stop worrying about what everyone else thinks or feels. Your ill child urgently needs you to be her advocate. More important, remember that most children with FMS get better after they reach adulthood!

Using medication

Low doses of mild antidepressants, such as Elavil (generic name: amitriptyline), that are administered in the evening may help your child with sleep difficulties and may also ease pain. However, the child may complain of feeling very sleepy in the morning with this medicine, and some children also complain of headaches.

Nonsteroidal anti-inflammatory drugs (NSAIDs), over-the-counter or prescribed, may be considered as well. These include over-the-counter drugs like ibuprofen and prescribed drugs like Vioxx (generic name: rofecoxib) or Celebrex (generic name: celecoxib).

Pediatricians report that NSAIDs usually are more effective with treating arthritis in children than they are with treating kids with juvenile fibromyalgia, although NSAIDs may give some relief to some children. The primary side effect that's identified with NSAIDs is stomach upset, and continued use of NSAIDs can result in *gastritis*, or stomach inflammation. (Read more about over-the-counter drugs for fibromyalgia in Chapter 9 and about prescribed medications for FMS in Chapter 10.)

Trying therapy

Because depression or anxiety often accompany fibromyalgia, the child or adolescent may benefit from receiving therapy as well as from taking antidepressants. As with adults, *cognitive-behavioral therapy* (CBT), which teaches the child how to challenge irrational or negative thoughts, is usually the most effective type of therapy.

A child psychologist can provide CBT. But a child psychiatrist is the most suitable professional to prescribe medications, such as antidepressants or anti-anxiety drugs as well as other medications used to treat emotional problems. Medical doctors who aren't psychiatrists can also prescribe medications, but they're not usually as knowledgeable about medications for emotional problems as are child psychiatrists.

Your child need not be mentally ill in order to see a child psychiatrist or psychologist. Psychiatrists and psychologists often see children with minor to major emotional problems, and depression is very common among children.

If you take your child with fibromyalgia to see a therapist, make sure that the therapist understands that the pain and symptoms of FMS are not solely created by a child's depression, anxiety, conflicts with parents or school, or other emotional issues. Symptoms may be worsened by such problems, but they don't cause the pain. If the therapist accepts that operating assumption, your child is more likely to succeed with the therapy that's provided.

Children up to the age of adolescence (and sometimes even teenagers!) may enjoy drawing a picture of Mr. Fibro as a way of communicating how they feel. After the child finishes the drawing, you and the child can briefly discuss Mr. Fibro. Don't deny his or her feelings, and let your child do most of the talking. (Adults tend to "jump in" before they're needed.)

Including Your Children Who Don't Have Fibromyalgia

When your child has a chronic medical problem, and it's one that your other child(ren) doesn't have, you may feel like you're doing a difficult balancing act sometimes. You don't want to pay so much attention to the sick child that the healthy children think that they have to act sick to be heard and seen. But at the same time, you can't ignore FMS, just as you can't ignore other chronic medical problems your child may have, such as diabetes, asthma, and so on.

Try to make sure that every child gets "special time" with you, tailoring the amount of time and the activity to the child. A teenager may need less time and may cringe in horror at the idea of going to a movie with a parent, and a younger child may love this idea. A walk may be a good idea instead. And explain that you don't love the sick child more or less than your other children. It's just that, sometimes, she or he needs a little extra help.

Working with Your Child's Teacher

One key arena where problems can crop up is in school. If your child is constantly saying that he or she can't do work or can't participate in gym, teachers may think that the child is "faking it." What should you do?

Should you tell your child's teacher that your daughter or son has fibromyalgia? You may think that the answer is an obvious *yes* (or, for that matter, an obvious *no*), but you have to consider some consequences that may occur, whatever you do (or don't do). Discussing the illness with the teacher is really an individual choice, but do keep in mind several factors:

- ✔ Teachers are prone to the same wrong ideas that are adopted by the general public. They may believe that fibromyalgia isn't a real illness or that it's something only adults can get.

- ✔ The teacher may treat your child differently — not in a good way — if she thinks that your child is disabled, making the workload too easy (or sometimes harder) for the child.

You want your child to get a good education and not be given a free pass. Yet, at the same time, you don't want your child to feel overwhelmed or physically ill from trying to reconcile her fibromyalgia symptoms with the demands of school. As a parent, you may find this path to be a tough one to navigate.

Children aren't allowed to bring any drugs to school, no matter how benign they may seem to you. Even bringing in an aspirin to school is usually strictly forbidden, and a child can be suspended or expelled for violating this policy. If your child needs to take medication during school hours, she's not alone. Bring a doctor's note or a prescription bottle with the child's name on it to school and explain to the school nurse what's needed. And don't worry. Many children have to take medicine during school.

Sharing information with teachers

If your child is missing a lot of school due to fibromyalgia, you may decide that you have to tell the teacher. Most schools have a limit of how many days can be missed before alarm bells go off in the school system, and someone, somewhere, may start to suspect that your child is "playing hooky" if he's missing many school days. You don't want to add allegations of truancy to your child's other problems.

If you do decide to tell your child's teacher about the fibromyalgia, consider the following points:

- ✔ Describe to the teacher what fibromyalgia is. She may never have heard of it. Explain to her that this is a problem that both adults and children can have and that the key symptoms are pain, fatigue, muscle stiffness, and sleep problems. And many children with FMS have frequent headaches as well.

- ✔ Tell the teacher that you don't want your child to avoid doing her schoolwork. If she can't handle the work during school time, ask if she can bring it home or if she can have a few days of extra time to complete the work.

✔ Offer to help ensure that your child completes her schoolwork. This offer may well present an extra burden on you, but it'll usually pay off in terms of obtaining cooperation and respect from your child's teacher.

✔ Explain to the teacher that you don't expect your child to be permanently excused from physical education. But on some days, although the child may be able to cope with her regular schoolwork, she won't be able to handle the demands of PE.

✔ If the teacher expresses doubt about fibromyalgia, don't flare up. Tell her that you can understand her concerns. But point out that in past years, many people didn't realize that children could suffer from ulcers, depression, and other medical problems. Tell her that FMS is a similar case.

✔ You can offer to share this book with the teacher (or buy her a copy), so that she can find out more about fibromyalgia. Point out this chapter to her. Sometimes, when people read information in a book, it has far more credibility than when you tell them the same thing.

Holding off on informing teachers

Maintaining a total nondisclosure policy about your child having an illness can become very difficult after awhile, and saying nothing usually isn't a good idea because teachers may think that your child has a worse problem than she has or that something terrible is occurring at home. But you may not want to share *every last detail* or even the exact diagnosis. So can you be partially forthcoming, without spilling all the beans? It's harder, but it's possible. Consider the following choices:

✔ Tell the teacher that your child has some medical problems that make it hard for her to concentrate right now. You're working on helping the child resolve these problems.

✔ Tell the teacher that your child has an illness that's similar to a mild form of arthritis.

✔ Ask the teacher to keep your information confidential. (Even when you've told her practically nothing.) Be sure to tell her whether she may (or may not) tell the other children or other teachers.

Not telling the teacher (or limiting what you tell him or her) has several benefits. Children are often embarrassed by information about them that's given by parents to teachers, especially if it can be considered negative. They may also fear being regarded as weak or disabled, and some teachers would possibly treat them that way if they knew about the fibromyalgia. Some teachers may also regard children with fibromyalgia as hypochondriacs, no matter how hard you work at educating them.

Handling difficult teachers

Sometimes, no matter how well you explain your child's problem and how helpful you try to be with the teacher, the situation deteriorates. The teacher starts telling others, including (worst case) other children about your child's medical problem. Or she doesn't believe that Susie is really sick, and she says so aloud to others. Other problems may also develop.

In such cases, the best thing to do is to ask for a meeting with the principal and the teacher to share your concerns. Don't be scared to ask for such a meeting! Write down the main one or two points you'd like to discuss at the meeting to make sure that you cover them. Plan ahead to be polite but firm.

Don't be intimidated, even if you're forced to sit in a little chair meant for a child. Your initial reaction, when you come to the meeting, may be to feel like *you've* been called to the principal's office. Remind yourself that you asked for this meeting.

Take notes in case the teacher or principal offers any good suggestions or agrees to some of your ideas. At the end of the meeting, summarize what you've agreed upon. "Okay, so my understanding is that Ms. Jones won't talk about Timmy's health to the other children anymore," or whatever it is.

Dealing with Jeers from Peers

One of the toughest "audiences" your child will have to face, whatever his or her problems, is that of the child's own peers. Children can be very cruel, taunting each other because they're fat (or skinny), wear glasses (or squint because they should wear glasses), are average (or are smart), and so on. When a child has a medical problem, such as fibromyalgia, kids may see this as just another thing to pick on. The child with fibromyalgia usually looks normal to others, but when they hang back from activities because of pain and fatigue, the other kids will notice.

Other children aren't necessarily mean or evil. (Although it may seem that way to the child who's being verbally attacked.) More often, the children are frustrated or upset about something else and take out their powerlessness on other children. However, it's not your job to analyze troubled children, but rather to help your own. And seeing their child unhappy is heartbreaking to parents. So what should you do? Here are a few suggestions, with the warning that they don't always work. Sadly, I can't offer you the one magic phrase that makes the blinders fall from the eyes of other children — or adults. But I hope they help.

If your child is verbally attacked

Most assaults aren't physical, but it's not true that "sticks and stones may break my bones, but names will never hurt me." Name-calling *does* hurt, and quite a lot. You may think that reasoning or explaining the fibromyalgia to the other child can help but, often, it doesn't. Name-calling is a power thing, not an understanding issue.

Of course, explaining that he or she has a disease that's like arthritis may help in some cases, so that's one way to go. Teach your child simple explanations of what fibromyalgia is — for example, that it's a medical problem that causes the body to hurt and get tired fast. Avoid complexities.

Sometimes, ignoring (or pretending to ignore) other children can help because they usually get bored or tired of the teasing. Most children have a fairly short attention span, and if the object of their bad attention seems unaffected, they'll move on to something or someone else.

If the teasing becomes constant and chronic and you sense that your child is being bullied, you can talk to the child who's doing the bullying yourself, if you can keep it nonthreatening and simple. You can also talk to the child's parents who may be horrified to find out about the verbal abuse. Some of them won't be, however. They may actually be part of the problem.

If your child is physically attacked

Sometimes, other children can become physically abusive, and taunting may escalate to pushing and even punching. If this type of violence happens to your child, it's illegal. Report it to the school authorities, if it happens at school, and if the abuse is beyond a few minor pushes, make sure that you also report it to the local police as well. Remind yourself that a bullying child who can be stopped and rehabilitated now is less likely to grow up to become an adult who assaults others. But above all, you need to protect your child from physical harm. That's part of your job as a parent.

Part VI
The Part of Tens

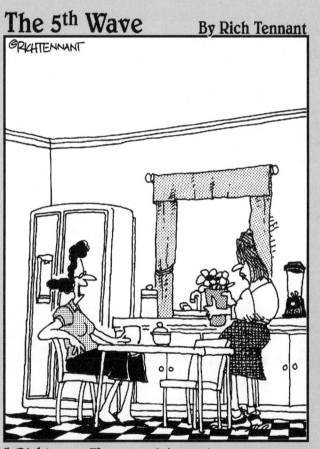

The 5th Wave   By Rich Tennant

@RICHTENNANT

" Right now I'm exercising pain management through medication, meditation, and limiting visits from my pain-in-the-butt neighbor. "

In this part . . .

What would a *For Dummies* book be without the famous Part of Tens? If you like quick and easy-to-read lists of things to do or not do, you'll love this part. Part VI provides ten different ways to explain fibromyalgia to others, ten "must-dos" when you have fibromyalgia, ten ways to cope with the confusion (*brain fog* or *fibro fog*) of fibromyalgia, and ten myths about this medical problem. I offer some valuable advice in this don't-miss part of the book.

Chapter 21

Ten Ways to Explain Fibromyalgia to Everyone (Even Your Doctor!)

• •

In This Chapter

▶ Providing frames of references to medical problems that others have

▶ Summarizing the painfulness, pervasiveness, and unpredictability of fibromyalgia

▶ Keeping in mind the knowledge and interest levels of the people you're talking to

• •

*B*ecause you're reading this book, you now know more about fibromyalgia syndrome (FMS) than most people, including some doctors! Bursting with knowledge, you may want to set the world straight on what fibromyalgia really is and how it affects you and others. Yet you can't instantly rectify the unawareness about fibromyalgia that's out there. But you *can* ease your own situation by conveying key points to friends, family members, and maybe even your own physician. In this chapter, I give you ten ways to explain fibromyalgia.

Chronically Speaking: How FMS Compares to Other Chronic Illnesses

Fibromyalgia is a chronic medical problem. And this fact is one way to explain it to others, so that they can relate to it better. A chronic disease is a continuing and serious medical problem that's not curable, but can be managed, like arthritis or thyroid disease. Chronic illness has ups and downs and requires medical treatment. Many people have a chronic illness or have a close relationship with someone who does. So most people know about chronic illness, up-close and personal.

Explain that in the case of FMS, the chronic problem is widespread muscular tenderness and pain that's usually accompanied by fatigue, sleep disorders, and other symptoms. Use other common chronic illnesses to explain the chronicity of FMS, such as:

✔ Hypertension (high blood pressure)

✔ Diabetes

✔ Chronic fatigue syndrome

In each of these illnesses, the medical problem requires careful monitoring and regular visits with doctors. None have any quick fixes, but their symptoms can improve with medications, exercise, and other remedies. The same is true for FMS.

Explaining the Pain

Pain is a major part of fibromyalgia, and it should be included in any explanation of FMS. Tell people, including physicians who haven't yet read up on the topic, that FMS is a medical problem in which the pain systems of the body have gone awry. Scientists aren't sure *why* the pain intensity is so great among people with FMS, but they do have some working theories, covered in more detail in Chapters 3 and 4. Here are some of these theories:

✔ The central nervous system has been sensitized to painful and non-painful events (Central Sensitization).

✔ Levels of Substance P (a pain neurochemical) are higher in people with FMS.

✔ Levels of cortisol and other hormones may be abnormal, increasing pain.

✔ People with FMS have impaired sleep patterns, which may cause or worsen their pain. (Sleep issues are also covered in Chapter 14.)

Gender-ly Speaking: Most People with FMS Are Female

Another way to explain fibromyalgia is to tell people that most victims are adult females — although men, adolescents, and children may have FMS, too. The reason that fibromyalgia predominates among women is unclear. Whether the illness is principally due to hormones or another cause is also unclear. Researchers are trying to find out why mostly women get FMS, and what they can do about it. However, assuming that men can't have FMS is a sexist attitude. Men with fibromyalgia can explain to others that, although it's true that most people with FMS are female, some sufferers are male, and you're one of them. (Gender issues are covered in more detail in Chapters 2 and 5.)

Accidentally Developing FMS

You can also talk about a possible cause, especially if it may apply to you. Some people with fibromyalgia have been involved in car crashes or other serious accidents before they developed fibromyalgia. Their systems may have become overstressed, and something may have triggered the hypersensitivity, pain, and fatigue that characterizes fibromyalgia. Most people can relate to and understand the after-effects of body trauma.

Affecting All Facets of Life

Another way to explain fibromyalgia to others is to emphasize that FMS plays a major role at work and at home, and that some people have to go on work disability because they're in so much pain and are so exhausted from this illness. They don't want to be sick, and they don't want to be deprived of interacting with people at work or at home, either. But fibromyalgia has a very pervasive effect on the lives of many people who have it.

Changing and Movable Areas of Pain

To truly educate others about fibromyalgia, be sure to tell them that many people have pain that moves from one part of the body to another. The intensity also often varies. Talk about the *tender points* of fibromyalgia, which are very sore when pressed. (You probably shouldn't tell them where *your* tender points are because some people may find it almost irresistible to touch or jab you on one of your areas of pain. "Does *this* hurt?")

Mentally Speaking

Fibromyalgia isn't caused by depression, anxiety, or any other emotional problems, but these problems often worsen FMS symptoms. Sometimes, having fibromyalgia can drive a person to depression because she may feel hopeless or helpless. Be sure to tell others that many chronic medical problems besides fibromyalgia, such as diabetes, hypertension, and arthritis, are also tied to depression or anxiety.

Unpredictably Yours, FMS

Another way to explain fibromyalgia is to tell people that the pain, fatigue, sleep loss, and other symptoms that are characteristic of FMS are *very unpredictable* in their severity. You never know whether to accept an invitation in advance because you may have to cancel it when the time comes, because of pain and exhaustion. Some people isolate themselves because they don't want to face the embarrassment of not showing up at the last minute. Tell others that if they can accept and understand the validity as well as the unpredictability of your problem, you're much more likely to be willing to make arrangements to meet with them.

Tailoring Your Explanation

You should always keep in mind the basic knowledge, interest level, and ability to understand of the people to whom you're explaining FMS. Don't "talk down" to people in a snotty way. But don't explain your fibromyalgia symptoms in the same way to your doctor as you would to your neighbor or your 10-year-old child. Choose your language to suit the level of understanding and interest of the person you're talking to. Most children won't comprehend explanations of Substance P, and most adults will want more information than just a statement that you hurt bad in a lot of places, frequently.

Comparing Past Non-Acceptance to Current Acceptance of Many Problems

You may also want to tell people that many other medical problems that weren't accepted in the past as valid, such as depression, headaches, or premenstrual syndrome (PMS), are now fully accepted by most people. Fibromyalgia isn't totally *there* yet, in terms of complete acceptance, but it's on its way. Tell people that, in the past, many people thought that individuals with depression were just trying to get attention or were lazy. Women with PMS were thought to be hysterical or trying to get out of work.

Fortunately, those old views are over for most people. Yet some people continue to mistakenly think that fibromyalgia is a fake problem. Tell the people that you're explaining FMS so that you know *they* aren't in the Dark Ages, and that they can understand and accept fibromyalgia as a valid problem. Verbally underline their enlightened attitude, whether you think it's there or not. Maybe you can help to create one.

Chapter 22

Ten Must-Dos for Everyone with Fibromyalgia

Maybe you can't follow every single bit of advice I offer you in this book. (Although I hope you consider trying many of my suggestions!) But do you think that you'd be able to sign up for at least ten "action items" to combat your fibromyalgia symptoms? If so, (and I hope that your answer is *yes*), read this chapter for a summation of ten must-dos when you have fibromyalgia syndrome (FMS). Try to do them all (but at least do some of them) to diminish your symptoms of fibromyalgia and improve how you feel.

Establishing a Good Working Relationship with Your Doctor

One of the most important must-do actions is to establish a good working relationship with your doctor. You need to have strong confidence in your doctor, and be willing to follow his or her advice. You also need a physician who listens to you, pays attention to the symptoms that you report, and partners with you to make a plan that you can (and will) follow. If you don't have such a relationship with your current doctor and you don't think that you can create one, read Chapter 7 about how to find a new physician.

Your doctor is important because he or she monitors and advises you on the following key elements of your FMS:

- ✔ Your overall symptoms (whether they're better, worse, or about the same)
- ✔ Medications you take (over-the-counter, prescribed medications, and alternative remedies)
- ✔ Lifestyle actions to take, tailored to your individual case (such as exercise recommendations, dietary advice, and so forth)

Listening to Your Body

Everyone who has fibromyalgia needs to "listen" to his or her body. You may say to yourself, "As if I *could* ignore it, it's screaming with pain at me." But I'm talking about a subtler kind of listening. Your body sends signals to you. And when you have FMS, you should respond to feeling overtired, overstressed, hungry, thirsty, or feeling a need to be alone, to name a few key signals that your body emits. In our busy society, many people try to ignore their body signals as long as possible. You shouldn't. If you give your body what it needs early on, you're more likely to improve your FMS symptoms.

De-Stressing Yourself As Much As Possible

Excessive stress is the problem that you need to work on, not "regular" stress. You can't possibly eliminate all stress from your life. Ridding all stress would also mean not enjoying the high points of life, such as the birth or adoption of a baby, a promotion at work, and many other joyous moments. The key is to keep your stress down to a workable level. Many people believe that large numbers of those individuals with fibromyalgia are high-achieving "Type A" kinds of people (although no research has been done on this belief). You can't change your genes or your personality if you're such a person, but you can scale down your expectations a little bit. Try the following suggestions:

- ✔ Use the "N" word: *No.* Don't take on more tasks than you can reasonably handle.
- ✔ Instead of demanding of yourself that you finish a job or project early, get it done on time. If you need more time, ask for it.
- ✔ Make sure that you give yourself some time off. Rest and relaxation is as important as sufficient sleep, a good diet, and enough exercise.
- ✔ Go for doing good work, but not perfection. Remember the old saying, "Better is the enemy of good enough."

Making Sure that You Sleep Enough Hours

Absolutely you must sleep at least seven hours per night because studies clearly show that a lack of sleep aggravates the symptoms of fibromyalgia. No, you don't have to act like a senior citizen and be in bed by 8 p.m. every night. But don't expect to stay up past midnight and then be bright and fresh at 6 a.m. the next day — especially day after day. Maybe you could do this when you were 16 (although doing so wasn't even advisable then). But now that you're an adult, and a person with FMS, treat your body right and get enough sleep.

Asking for What You Need From Others

Many people with FMS seem to be afraid or embarrassed to tell others what they need, whether it's help with specific tasks, some time off from work because of being exhausted and overwhelmed, or just to be left alone for awhile. Telling others what you need is perfectly okay. (At the same time, never take advantage of your FMS to get out of things you'd rather not do even when you feel okay, such as taking out the trash, cleaning the toilet, or other tasks that you hate.) People may not always *give* you what you ask for, but if you don't ask, you'll never know. So, ask.

Avoiding Overdoing It on Good Days

Because you feel so bad on really bad days, you may feel the need to try to cram as many activities as possible into days when you feel less awful or even close to normal. The problem with that policy is that if you overwork yourself on better days, payback later can be painful. Pace yourself as much as possible. It'll usually be worth it, in terms of giving yourself fewer bad days.

Maintaining a Positive Attitude

When you feel really bad, maintaining a positive mental attitude can be tough. But many people with fibromyalgia say that if they can joke about the problem — even in a sort of sarcastic, crabby way — it can help to ease the pain, at least a little. It may sound silly, and a bit like that old movie *Annie,* but try this: Tell yourself that tomorrow will be a better day. Also, try smiling, even if it feels like the most fake and insincere act you can imagine. It doesn't always work but, sometimes, acting happy (even when you start out by faking it) can actually make you feel better. It may take some time, but the pain will get better!

Coping with Depression

Many people with fibromyalgia do become depressed, which is a worse situation than mere sadness. Depression's also something that you can't fix by pasting a smile on your face. (Although the smile tactic is usually worth a try.) Fibromyalgia may cause people to become depressed, or FMS and depression may simply go together somehow, biochemically. If you're experiencing depression and the usual things that cheer you up don't come close to working, see a therapist and get some help. Depression is highly treatable with medication and/or talking with a good therapist.

Working with Family and Friends

Whether you realize it or not, your family and friends are deeply affected by your fibromyalgia. Ignoring this fact won't make it go away. The best approach is to talk to your family and friends about what you can and can't do and to give them a mini-education on fibromyalgia. Of course, you shouldn't drone on endlessly about FMS, or they'll tune you out. Also, keep in mind that fibromyalgia is nobody's fault. It's not your fault, and it's not your family's or friends' fault. It just exists. It's like having arthritis, diabetes, or high blood pressure. Sure, people can make you feel worse by making demands or yelling at you. But the fact remains that they don't cause the problem in the first place. Make sure that they know this. How? Tell them. (I give you tips on explaining your FMS to family and friends in Chapter 18.)

Handling Work (Or NOT Handling Work, if You Need to Stop Working)

If you're working full-time or part-time and your fibromyalgia is making your work life an impossible situation, you need to make some changes. Maybe you can make some simple changes at work, such as taking more breaks or asking for a more comfortable chair. Or maybe you need to make bigger changes, such as working fewer hours, working from home, going from full-time work to part-time work, or going to another job altogether.

In some cases, you should face facts and realize that your illness is preventing you from doing the good job that you want and need to do. There's no shame or dishonor in taking time off or even applying for a disability when you just can't do your job anymore.

Chapter 23

Ten Ways to Beat the Effects of Brain Fog

In This Chapter

▶ Overcoming your mental malaise (otherwise known as brain fog)

▶ Defining the important tasks

▶ Working with others to help you stay on task

*L*aurie says that the forgetfulness, confusion, and overall *brain fog* that seem to go together with fibromyalgia syndrome (FMS) really drive her crazy, and she'd love some helpful hints on how to pull herself together when she starts lapsing into la-la land. What she'd really like is for the brain fog (and the fibromyalgia) to evaporate like a morning mist, except forever (mist comes back the next day). Barring that, some coping techniques are her order of the day.

This chapter offers Laurie (and you) some basic guidelines on ways to stay present and focused in the here and now and to achieve most (if not all) of what you need to get done. If brain fog washes over you anyway, which often happens, these techniques can help you to maintain some semblance of order in your life. In this chapter, I offer ten basic helpful hints for beating back your brain fog or averting the effects when you can't avoid it.

Avoiding Brain and Energy Drains When You're Hurting or Tired

This piece of advice may sound like a "no-brainer," but I'll say it anyway: You really shouldn't try to tackle difficult problems when your symptoms are in the red (very high) zone of pain. Yet many people feel that they must *still* help their child with a complicated science project, drive five hours to a family reunion, or perform some other difficult task that requires more brain power and energy than you can reasonably give when you're in pain. Is it any wonder, in such cases, that you become confused and a little foggy?

Think of your mind and body as like a glass of water, full to the brim with your active life. Then imagine trying to add *more* water (work) to the glass because you think that you should. You get a mess that spills over into your personal and professional lives. Also, while you're struggling to take on the big jobs, you may be ignoring easy and doable tasks that are still within your capabilities, such as work or household tasks that need to be done.

The best policy is to keep it simple when you're sick. If you do, you'll be far more likely to avoid forgetfulness and confusion and to stay focused. If you really *must* do something hard (and are you sure about the "must" part?), try to break it down into smaller tasks, doing some now and some later.

Asking Others to Help You Stay On Task

If you're periodically short-circuiting in terms of mental alertness because of your FMS symptoms, consider making an ally at work or at home who can help you come back to Planet Earth. Ask this person to notice if you seem to be "lost in space," brainwise, and to send you a signal. The signal can be a gentle touch on the arm, a word or phrase that grabs your attention, or something else.

Of course, any previously agreed-upon cue should also be something that avoids embarrassment to your friend. Standing on his head may work well to get your attention, but other people may wonder whether your friend needs professional help. You can also try a more general approach of telling people that, sometimes, you get lost in thought and, if you seem inattentive, to please call on you by name more loudly than usual. (No screaming allowed.)

Making Lists and Checking Them Twice

Listmaking is an efficient procedure for most busy people, and it can really help a person constrained by fibromyalgia. The only downside of lists is that many people tend to be overly ambitious about what they can perform in a day or a week. Write down what you absolutely must do today, and then prioritize the items from most important down to the least important. (Don't make your first task a nearly impossible one.)

A list can help you focus. And if you're having a bad day, often you'll still have succeeded at doing at least a few things on your list, and can pat yourself on the back. No name-calling of yourself, however, if you can't accomplish your list items. Nobody's perfect.

Banning Self-Blame

Many people become inordinately angry with themselves when they're sick and can't remember to do things (or simply *can't* do them, even if they do remember them). Don't make this mistake because you're likely to worsen your brain fog further if you cloud up you mind with negative self-talk. Does anyone work better when they're being yelled at? It may work if you're joining the Marines, but for most people, being yelled at makes them more confused. Don't chastise yourself, either. Do the best you can and let the rest go until tomorrow.

Avoiding Blaming Others

In addition to a tendency to blame yourself for not doing everything you think that you should be doing, sometimes, when you're sick, you may find yourself blaming others for not making your life sufficiently easy. Whether you self-blame or blame others, you're likely to worsen your fibro fog. Avoid this problem. Don't let others get away with not doing what they're supposed to at home or at work. But don't blame them because you feel lousy. It's not their fault. (Or yours.)

Getting Enough Sleep

I emphasize the importance of obtaining enough sleep in other chapters throughout the book, and guess what? Here it is again. Sufficient sleep (at least seven hours a night) is vitally important for the brain and the body. You concentrate better and think more clearly when you have thoroughly rested your entire body through the process known as sleep. If you don't get enough sleep, however, you'll find it much harder to wrap your mind around even the simplest of concepts — let alone concentrate on serious issues. Get the rest you need on a regular basis, and often, the fibro fog will clear up.

Keeping a Calendar of Activities

Making lists is a good idea, and another good idea is to keep a calendar of what you're supposed to do and when. On a day when you're not over-whelmed with symptoms, you should record doctor's appointments, birthdays, and other important dates and activities that you really need to pay attention to on your calendar. Forget relying on those little cards doctors give people. You can easily lose them or forget about them altogether. Instead, when you get home from a doctor's appointment, immediately write down the dates and times in your calendar.

Watching What You Eat

How on earth can the foods that you *eat* affect your brain's performance? Simply put, some foods can impair productivity, making you more sluggish. Others make sleeping more difficult. (And some foods, such as turkey or milk, can help you fall asleep.) Read more about good foods/bad foods in Chapter 15. The following foods can worsen brain fog:

- ✔ Caffeine, such as in soft drinks, tea, coffee, and chocolate (these foods hype you up, making it hard for you to sleep)

- ✔ Excessive sugar can make you tired and cranky — definitely *not* good for brain fog.

- ✔ Foods that contain additives, such as MSG, can cause agitation. Avoid them.

Putting Things in Their Places

If you're distracted by your symptoms and are prone to misplacing things like your car keys and important papers, you need to adopt an aggressive policy of putting the most important items in the same places over and over. Concentrate on the two or three most important items you need, but which you keep losing in your fibro fog. For many people, car keys are a biggie. Some people place their car keys on a ring by the door, and others put them in a particular place in their purse or pants pocket. If you always put the item in the same place, you're more likely to avoid wasting your time searching for items you need when you're feeling major pain.

Catching Yourself Slipping Away

It may sound unlikely, but you can actually catch yourself in the act of slipping into a brain fog. Some people with a frequent brain fog problem use visual or auditory signals, such as an alarm that goes off every half-hour or hour. Even using a screen saver on your computer may help because if you're staring at the screen, you'll probably notice when all goes black. You can buy special watches that beep or pulsate at preprogrammed intervals, bringing you back to the world of the self-aware. Do realize, however, that everyone daydreams or tunes out the world sometimes, and doing so can be a good thing, once in awhile.

Chapter 24

Ten Myths about Fibromyalgia

. . . .

In This Chapter

▶ Mastering the myths and realities of fibromyalgia

▶ Helping others understand what's real and not real

▶ Maintaining perspective

. . . .

I talk about some of the fibromyalgia myths in other chapters throughout this book. Some of these myths say that fibromyalgia is imaginary, and people who think they've got it are either lazy or crazy. Another myth is that people who say that they have fibromyalgia syndrome (FMS) are really drug or attention seekers. Of course, you've probably heard of many more myths that you could describe on your own. Plenty of myth-busting needs to be done when it comes to fibromyalgia. I believe that knowledge is power, and after you understand what's most important to know about fibromyalgia from your own perspective, you may want to share this information with others and empower them, too.

In this chapter, I cover ten key myths about fibromyalgia and explain why these myths aren't valid. You'll probably recognize at least some of these myths, and you may get an "Aha!" reaction with all or most of them.

People with Fibromyalgia Are Lazy or Crazy

One of the most common myths about fibromyalgia is that it's an escape clause for people who don't feel like working or who are so emotionally disturbed that they imagine that they're sick. The "lazy or crazy" myth is even believed by a few doctors, although most physicians know that it isn't true. Studies indicate that people with FMS are as active as people who don't have fibromyalgia, *except* when they're in the middle of a major flare-up of pain and fatigue.

It only makes sense: When you feel really sick, you can't work as well as usual, or maybe you can't work at all. A truly "lazy" person is physically fit, but he or she prefers to do nothing.

Nor are people with fibromyalgia delusional about their symptoms. What they feel is real, and is no figment of the imagination. Many people with fibromyalgia *do* suffer from problems with depression (covered in Chapter 2), anxiety, and stress (covered in Chapter 13). But none of these problems makes them develop FMS. Something else causes fibromyalgia.

Fibromyalgia Symptoms Are a Way to Get Attention

Another myth that drives people with fibromyalgia wild is that they're "just trying to get attention." Patients with FMS agree that they'd rather be in solitary confinement than to suffer a severe flare-up of fibromyalgia. Their suffering is in no way an attempt to get center stage with their friends and relatives.

People with FMS Just Want Drugs

Because many people with fibromyalgia need painkilling medications at least some of the time, some people may assume that people with FMS are really "druggies" who are seeking an excuse to take strong painkillers or narcotics. Although some painkilling drugs *can* be habit forming and need close monitoring by physicians, people who take drugs for pain rather than to get high have a lowered risk of becoming addicted to drugs.

Looking Well Means You ARE Well

Charlotte was always well dressed, and her general demeanor gave no indication of any of the pain that she suffered from fibromyalgia. If you were to look *really* closely, though, you may you sometimes see an almost imperceptible tightness around the mouth and eyes. You may also notice that Charlotte didn't smile a lot and rarely laughed. People thought that Charlotte was a distant kind of person, but the reality was that she suffered from fibromyalgia. When people told her how well she looked, she always thought, "If they only knew!"

Some illnesses aren't readily apparent from the "outside," and fibromyalgia is one of them — along with diabetes, hypertension (or high blood pressure), and mild arthritis. Most people who have such medical problems may be told that they look wonderful, even when they don't go to great lengths to hide their illness, like Charlotte. Telling someone that you feel awful only to hear in response, "But you look so great!" can be truly maddening. Remember (and tell your friends): Looking wonderful may be the same as feeling wonderful. But when you have fibromyalgia, that often isn't the case.

Pain is Pain: It's All the Same

All pain is not created equal. If your cousin has pain from arthritis or a bad back, she may think that her pain is about the same as your pain from fibromyalgia. (Or she may think that her pain is worse!) But studies indicate that the pain from fibromyalgia can be more intense than other forms of muscle or joint pain, and it often lasts longer as well.

Feeling Good Today Means You're Well

Fibromyalgia is a frustrating kind of disease because it can be so unpredictable. Today, you feel lousy; tomorrow, you feel worse; the next day, you feel okay or even close to normal. When you tell people that you're having a good day, many will assume that you're "all better." People often have a hard time grasping a medical problem that has a lot of ups and downs to it. But that's the nature of the illness.

Relaxing Will Cure What Ails You

When your symptoms from FMS are really bothering you, a lot of people will tell you that you're working too hard, that you need to ease off. They may advise you that a week on a cruise or a nice vacation to a pleasant place will fix you right up. In fact, you *may* be working too hard right now, and stress certainly can exacerbate fibromyalgia. Maybe some rest and relaxation would make you feel much better. But when you have fibromyalgia, a vacation can't cure you. You could win the lottery and retire tomorrow, and you'd still have periodic flare-ups of the problem.

Taking Some Pills Will Fix You

Some people become annoyed when you tell them about your pain and advise you to "take a pill," whether it's Tylenol, Prozac, or something else. Many people are very drug oriented in our society. This can be good in that people are willing to take medications that can help them, and a great many medications are available to treat fibromyalgia. But assuming that swallowing a few pills will completely resolve your problem is not good. Medications are short-term fixes for the long-term problem of fibromyalgia. (I discuss over-the-counter and prescription medications in Chapters 9 and 10.)

Ignoring the Problem Will Make It Go Away

Your partner or your friends may tell you that you're dwelling on your symptoms too much. Distract yourself, think about something else, and you'll feel better. To a certain extent, if you're able to distract yourself with interesting work or family tasks, you may be able to ignore some of the pain. But most of it will still be there, whether you try to ignore it or not.

Therapy Always Works

Some people think that the answer to any long-term problem is therapy, and that a good therapist can help you work through all your problems. Although a therapist can certainly help you if you have problems with anxiety, depression, or stress, that therapist can't cure your fibromyalgia. You probably will feel *some* better after talking to a therapist — but not *all* better.

Part VII
Appendixes

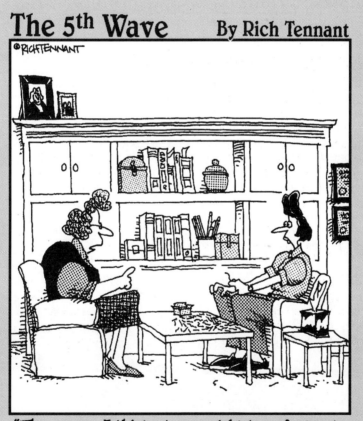

The 5th Wave   By Rich Tennant

"The reason I think stress might be a factor in your FMS is because of research, statistics, and the fact that you've straightened out an entire box of paper clips during our conversation."

In this part . . .

The last part of this book includes appendixes. I offer
you a glossary of terms, so you can easily look up
the definitions for key fibromyalgia-related words. I also
provide a very helpful list of medications, both over-the-
counter and prescribed drugs, which are often recommended to people with fibromyalgia. You may know these
medications by their brand name or their "generic" name,
so I give you both, along with the main side effects that
the medications may cause.

If you wish to uncover even more information on fibromyalgia after you've finished reading this book, check
out my appendix of important resources that includes
organizations with helpful information, publications that
may intrigue you, and Internet sources for fibromyalgia-
related info.

Appendix A

Glossary

• •

*I*n this appendix, I provide brief definitions of some major terms used throughout this book that are important for people with fibromyalgia syndrome (FMS) to understand (as well as others who are interested in FMS).

acupuncture: Insertion of tiny needles into distinct muscle areas to stimulate the production of *endorphins* (natural painkilling biochemicals). Scientists at the National Institutes of Health (NIH) are currently evaluating the success of acupuncture in treating fibromyalgia and other medical problems.

alternative medicine: Treatments or medications that are not viewed as traditional and have not undergone a rigorous scientific evaluation. Alternative medicine includes the use of herbal and mineral supplements and acupuncture, as well as other remedies and treatments.

arthritis: An illness that affects the joints of the body. Many people with lupus and rheumatoid arthritis have joint pain and inflammation.

Arthritis Foundation: Nonprofit organization that provides information on fibromyalgia and arthritis to consumers and medical professionals and also funds key clinical studies on both fibromyalgia and arthritis.

botox injections: Injections of minute amounts of botulinum toxins into the muscles and other areas of the body where patients feel pain. This is a controversial and costly treatment, and its use in fibromyalgia is not yet approved by the Food and Drug Administration (FDA).

chronic fatigue syndrome (CFS): Medical problem that's primarily characterized by extreme exhaustion and pain, and that is often confused with fibromyalgia.

cortisol: A stress related hormone that's been found in abnormal levels in some people who have fibromyalgia.

depression: Serious form of despair that's beyond the normal feelings of sadness. Many people with fibromyalgia suffer from depression, but it is highly treatable.

dextromethorphan: Medication that is commonly used to treat coughs. Some research has indicated dextromethorphan may provide some pain relief in fibromyalgia.

fibro fog: Mental confusion and forgetfulness that can accompany a flare-up of fibromyalgia symptoms. Also known as *brain fog*.

fibromyalgia: Chronic pain condition that is characterized by ***tender points*** (see definition later in this appendix), widespread pain, morning stiffness, sleep disturbances, and distress.

guaifenesin: Drug commonly used to treat coughs, which is also used by some physicians to treat fibromyalgia. Studies have not validated this use.

Gulf War syndrome: Condition characterized by fatigue and widespread pain and body aches related to active duty in the 1991 Persian Gulf war. Some Gulf War veterans also have fibromyalgia, and they may be eligible for compensation from the Veterans Administration.

headaches, tension or migraine: Head pain that is either related to muscle tension or migraine attacks, two specific forms of headaches. Many people with fibromyalgia also suffer from headaches.

heartburn: Chronic pain and burning in the gut that often results from gastroesophageal reflux. Stomach acid backs up into the esophagus and causes pain. Many people with fibromyalgia also have heartburn.

icing or heating therapy: Refers to therapy in which the painful areas of the body are stimulated through treatments with either ice or heat (such as a heating pad). Icing and heating are usually effective methods of treating fibromyalgia.

interstitial cystitis (IC): Chronic illness of pain with urination and increased urgency. Some people with fibromyalgia also suffer from IC.

irritable bowel syndrome (IBS): Chronic condition that is often characterized by abdominal pain in conjunction with constipation and/or diarrhea. Some people with fibromyalgia also suffer from IBS.

Lyme disease: Bacterial illness spread by a tick, which can cause severe tiredness. A blood test can confirm the presence of Lyme disease. In diagnosis, Lyme disease may be confused with fibromyalgia.

massage therapy: A form of treatment in which painful areas of the body are gently rubbed to help with pain management. Massage therapy can be helpful in treating fibromyalgia.

mononucleosis: Infectious disease that can cause extreme lethargy, which may be confused with fibromyalgia; however, mononucleosis can be diagnosed with a blood test.

multiple chemical sensitivities syndrome (MCSS): A condition in which the person has become extremely sensitive to many substances that were never a problem before, such as odors, foods, and common items.

myofascial pain syndrome: A condition characterized by regional pain as well as by local areas of pain (called *trigger points*) that the doctor can identify upon touching them. In contrast, the ***tender points*** (see definition later in this appendix) of fibromyalgia cannot be felt by doctors.

oligoanalgesia: The undertreatment, ineffectual treatment, or lack of treatment of pain. Some patients with fibromyalgia have this problem until they find a good physician.

pain diary: Written record of when pain is most severe, which helps patients track conditions that may trigger pain, such as foods or other items.

painkilling medications: Over-the-counter or prescribed medications taken to reduce pain from fibromyalgia.

pain management: Controlling chronic pain to a tolerable level, with medications, massage therapy, physical therapy, and other treatments.

physiatrist: Another type of doctor who treats fibromyalgia in addition to the rheumatologist. Also known as a 'sports medicine' doctor.

post-traumatic stress disorder (PTSD): A hyper-aroused state arising from extreme stress, which may continue long after the distressing incident occurred. People who suffer from PTSD may develop physical symptoms immediately after the incident (or six months or more later) that lead to fibromyalgia.

reflex sympathetic dystrophy (RSD): A serious and painful condition that is most frequently found in the patient's arms or legs. It may be confused with fibromyalgia, in some cases.

relaxation therapy: Technique that allows a person under extreme stress to decrease stress levels. Lowering high levels of stress usually improves the symptoms of a person with fibromyalgia.

rheumatologist: Physician who specializes in treating arthritis, autoimmune diseases, and fibromyalgia.

sleep disorders: Difficulty in getting to sleep and/or staying asleep. Sleep disorders are extremely common among people with fibromyalgia.

Social Security disability compensation: Monthly compensation and medical insurance (Medicare) provided by the Social Security Administration to eligible individuals who cannot work because of fibromyalgia or other medical problems. Individuals must apply to be considered.

Substance P: A neurochemical whose levels have been shown to be higher in patients with fibromyalgia.

supplements: Minerals or herbs that may provide relief to people with fibromyalgia. Some research has indicated that supplemental magnesium is helpful to some patients with fibromyaglia.

T'ai Chi: Chinese exercise technique that mimics the movements of animals. T'ai Chi is not a physically aggressive form of exercise, and most people with fibromyalgia can tolerate performing these exercises.

tender points: Specific areas of the body that are painful when touched if a person has fibromyalgia. People with FMS generally have pain in at least 11 of the 18 specific tender point sites.

thyroid disease: Malfunction of the thyroid gland that results in either abnormally high or low levels of circulating thyroid hormone. This disease may result in symptoms that can be confused with fibromyalgia and other illnesses.

Appendix B

Fibromyalgia Medications

● ●

*I*n this appendix, I provide you with listings of both prescribed and over-the counter-medications that may be recommended to you and other people with fibromyalgia syndrome (FMS). I include the following information: the brand name of the drug, the generic name, and the primary side effects that may occur, although side effects aren't experienced by everyone. (In a few cases, the brand name and the generic name are the same, as with guaifenesin and dextromethorphan.)

I provide these listings for your information only, and you should not in any way consider this information to be any sort of a substitute for consulting with your own physician and following his or her medical recommendations.

Pondering Prescribed Medications

Whether you have severe pain, fatigue, and/or sleep problems from your fibromyalgia or just minor discomfort, at some point, you will need prescription drugs to treat your FMS symptoms. You may need to take meds on a regular basis, or you may only need to take them when your symptoms flare up. Whatever your needs, here's some information about the different types of prescription medications that are prescribed for fibromyalgia.

Sometimes, anti-anxiety medications can help with the pain generated by fibromyalgia as well as with the sleep problems that many people with FMS suffer from. All anti-anxiety drugs listed in Table B-1 may be sedating and may cause nightmares. Xanax may be especially habit forming.

Table B-1	Anti-Anxiety Medications
Brand Name	*Generic Name*
Klonopin	Clonazepam
Librium	Chlordiazepoxide
Restoril	Temazepam
Valium	Diazepam
Xanax	Alprazolam

Often, antidepressants are prescribed for people with fibromyalgia because they can help with the pain and the insomnia experienced by most people with FMS. Antidepressants (listed in Table B-2) may be sedating, and they may also cause weight gain or loss and stomach upset. Prozac may cause a loss of libido.

Table B-2	Antidepressants
Brand Name	*Generic Name*
Adapin	Doxepin
Effexor	Venlafaxine
Elavil	Amitriptyline
Pamelor	Nortriptyline
Paxil	Paroxetine
Prozac	Fluoxetine
Zoloft	Sertraline

Anti-epileptic medications can sometimes provide relief from pain and muscle aches experienced by people with fibromyalgia. All anti-epileptic medications listed in Table B-3 may be sedating and may cause dry mouth or dizziness.

Table B-3	Anti-Epileptic Medications
Brand Name	*Generic Name*
Lamictal	Lamotrigine
Neurontin	Gabapentin
Topamax	Topiramate

Muscle relaxants are often prescribed for people with fibromyalgia, because they can offer some relief from muscle aches and pains. They're usually taken at night because they can make you sleepy, too. All muscle relaxants listed in Table B-4 may cause sedation, diarrhea, and stomach pain.

Table B-4	**Muscle Relaxants**
Brand Name	*Generic Name*
Baclofen	Baclofen
Flexeril	Cyclobenzaprine
Norflex	orphenadrine citrate
Soma	Carisoprodol
Skelaxin	Metaxalone
Zanaflex	tizanidine HCl

Nonsteroidal anti-inflammatory drugs (NSAIDs) are prescribed for pain relief. All NSAIDs listed in Table B-5 may cause gastrointestinal pain and bleeding and diarrhea. "Coxib" (Cox 2) drugs, such as Bextra, Celebrex, and Vioxx, have a lower risk of gastrointestinal problems.

Table B-5	**Nonsteroidal Anti-Inflammatory Drugs (NSAIDs)**
Brand Name	*Generic Name*
Bextra	Valdecoxib
Celebrex	Celecoxib
Feldene	Piroxicam
Naprosyn	naproxen sodium
Relafen	Nabumetone
Vioxx	Rofecoxib

People with FMS often suffer from major pain, and they need a drug that's specifically meant to combat pain symptoms. Painkillers are usually sedating, and some, such as Demerol, OxyContin, Perodan, Percocet, and Vicodin, can be habit forming.

Table B-6	Painkillers	
Brand Name	*Generic Name*	*Comments*
Demerol	Meperidine	A narcotic, sedating, habit-forming
Fiorcet	Butalbital, acetaminophen	Sedating
OxyContin	Oxycodone	A narcotic, sedating, habit-forming
Percocet	Oxycodone with acetaminophen	Sedating, habit-forming
Percodan	Oxycodone with aspirin	Sedating, habit-forming
Tylenol 3	Acetaminophen with codeine	Sedating, constipating, habit-forming
Ultracet	Tramadol with acetaminophen	Sedating, habit-forming
Ultram	Tramadol	Sedating, habit-forming
Vicodin	Hydrocodone	Sedating, habit-forming

Most people with fibromyalgia struggle with getting to sleep, and sometimes, nothing seems to work. As a result, doctors may prescribe sleep remedies. The sleep medications listed in Table B-7 may cause continued sedation. Ambien may cause diarrhea. Desyrel may cause weight gain.

Table B-7	Sleep Medications
Brand Name	*Generic Name*
Ambien	Zolpidem
Desyrel	Trazodone
Sonata	Zaleplon

Reviewing Over-the-Counter Medications

Over-the-counter (OTC) drugs are often recommended to patients with fibromyalgia because they can help relieve pain and sleep problems. Of course, just because a drug isn't prescribed doesn't mean that it's automatically safe or that it will help you. Every medication has side effects that you should consider before taking the drug.

Some physicians may recommend cold remedies to help alleviate some of your FMS symptoms. Cold remedies, such as the ones listed in Table B-8, cause few side effects but some, such as Delsym, may be sedating. Others, such as dextromethorphan or guaifenesin, can cause itchy skin and rashes in some people.

Table B-8	Cough/Cold Remedies	
Brand Name	*Generic Name*	*Comments*
Delsym	dextromethorphan polistirex	Includes alcohol, may be sedating
Dextromethorphan	dextromethorphan	May cause Itching, rashes
Guaifenesin	guaifenesin	May cause Itching, rashes

You may not want or need a prescribed drug to deal with your pain, and common OTC painkillers (like the ones listed in Table B-9) may do the job just fine. Their side effects vary and can be serious; for example, if you're constantly taking Tylenol, you risk liver damage, and it may be better to switch to another OTC drug or a prescribed medication.

Table B-9	Painkillers	
Brand Name	*Generic Name*	*Comments*
Aleve	naproxen potassium	May cause headaches, ringing in the ears, stomach ulcers.
Aspirin	acetyl-salicylate	May cause easy bruising, gastrointestinal bleeding.
Motrin	ibuprofen	May cause nausea, stomach upset, stomach ulcers.
Tylenol	Acetaminophen	Excessive use can damage liver; alcohol should be avoided with this drug.

There are many topical (applied to your skin) remedies for pain. In fact, so many topical remedies are available that I can't possibly list a fair assortment of them here. Topical remedies do have some common denominators, however. Nearly all contain one or more of the following ingredients, and topical remedies may cause burning or numbness.

- ✔ Capsaicin (from chili peppers)
- ✔ Cayenne (also from chili peppers)
- ✔ Eucalyptus
- ✔ Methyl salicylate (from aspirin)
- ✔ Menthol
- ✔ Peppermint oil

Appendix C

Resources and Support

*I*n this appendix, I provide you with lists of organizations and Internet resources that may be of interest to people with fibromyalgia syndrome (FMS), as well as to their family and friends. I don't personally endorse any of these listings (nor does the publisher), and I'm not responsible for their content, but I hope that you find them useful and helpful.

Organizations

National and international organizations throughout the United States, Canada, the United Kingdom, and other countries provide a wealth of information, educational materials, and morale-boosting offerings. Most of these organizations also provide newsletters, brochures, and other publications. (Some of the publications are free, and some items are available for a fee.) Here's a rundown on some key groups with an interest in fibromyalgia:

- American Chronic Pain Association (ACPA), P.O. Box 850, Rocklin, CA 95677; Phone: 800-533-3231; Internet: www.theacpa.org.

- Arthritis Foundation, P.O. Box 7669, Atlanta, GA 30357; Phone: 800-283-7800; Internet: www.arthritis.org.

- The Arthritis Society, 393 University Avenue, Suite 1700, Toronto, Ontario, M5G 1E6, Canada; Phone: 416-979-7228 or toll-free: 800-321-1433; Internet: www.arthritis.ca.

- CFIDS Association of America, Inc., P.O. Box 20398, Charlotte, NC 28222; Phone: 800-442-3437; Internet: www.cfids.org.

- Fibromyalgia Association UK, P.O. Box 206, Stourbridge, DY9 8YL; Phone 0870-752-5118; Internet: www.fibromyalgia-associationuk.org.

- National Center for Complementary and Alternative Medicine (NCCAM) Clearinghouse, P.O. Box 8218, Silver Spring, MD 20907; Phone: 888-644-6226; Internet: www.nccam.nih.gov.

- National Institute of Arthritis and Musculoskeletal and Skin Diseases (NIAMS) Clearinghouse, 1 AMS Circle, Bethesda, MD 20892; Phone: 877-226-4267; Internet: www.nih.gov/niams.

To find local support groups interested in fibromyalgia, ask your local reference librarian for help (not the librarian at the front desk, but the one who works at the reference section of the library.) Also, ask your doctors who treat fibromyalgia and any friends or relatives who have fibromyalgia if they know of any local groups.

Finding Information on the Internet

The Internet has a variety of options available that provide opportunities to gain information and share what you know about fibromyalgia and meet other people with similar interests. The key formats of these options are Web sites, e-mail lists, newsgroups, and forums.

Spotting the frauds, scams, and just plain crazy ideas on the Internet isn't always easy. But it's often possible. Keep a few basics in mind. First, try to determine who's running the Web site by locating the "contact us" or similar icon or looking on the main page. If you can't find such an icon and no matter how hard you look, you can't find a name, mailing address, and a telephone number, alarm bells should ring. They're saying: Don't buy anything with your credit card from these people.

Another screening tactic is to try to determine the primary purpose of this site. Is it an information-only site, or are you bombarded with offers to buy this and that wonder-cure? If so, watch out. And speaking of wonder cures, if you're offered a quickie and forever cure, run away. Sorry, but it isn't that easy.

If you're still not sure whether you should buy a product that you're told you need RIGHT NOW!, try this: Imagine that the site was offering products for another medical problem, one you don't have, such as diabetes or asthma. Would the offers still seem credible? If not, say goodbye.

Checking out Web sites that may appeal

Hundreds of different Web sites on the Internet have either a direct or indirect concentration on the subject of fibromyalgia. Some popular sites include the following:

- American Academy of Rheumatology, fibromyalgia information (www.rheumatology.org/patients/factsheet/fibromya.html)
- American Fibromyalgia Syndrome Association, Inc. (www.afsafund.org)
- Arthritis Foundation, fibromyalgia resources (www.arthritis.org)

- Fibrohugs Fibromyalgia Support Site (www.fibrohugs.com)

- Fibromyalgia Network (www.fmnetnews.com)

- Fibromyalgia Resource Center (www.healingwell.com/fibro)

- MEDLINEplus, fibromyalgia (www.nlm.nih.gov/medlineplus/fibromyalgia.html)

- Missouri Arthritis Rehabilitation Research and Training Center (www.hsc.missouri.edu/~fibro/index.html)

- National Fibromyalgia Association (www.fmaware.org)

- National Fibromyalgia Research Association (www.nfra.net)

- Oregon Fibromyalgia Foundation (www.myalgia.com)

- University of Florida Fibromyalgia Research Information (www.med.ufl.edu/rheum/)

Looking at e-mail lists

An e-mail list, also called a *listserv,* is an arrangement whereby you join as a member and automatically receive all e-mails sent by every member. (Sometimes, e-mail lists provide you the option of going to a special Web site to read all the messages if you don't want to receive a large number of e-mails.)

Before joining an e-mail list, consider the pros and cons of doing so. Here are some of the positive aspects of joining e-mail lists:

- You may gain information that's difficult or impossible to obtain elsewhere. (Some *posters,* people who send e-mail to the list participants, are medical professionals.)

- You may feel a strong kinship to others who are going through problems that you are facing.

As with almost everything in this world, e-mail lists also have a few strikes against them:

- You must wade through a large number of responses. An active list can generate many messages! My coauthor told me that she joined a listserv once and received 100 messages the first day and even more the second day! On the third day, she begged to be removed from the list because she just couldn't keep up. Not all listservs are overwhelmingly active, but some are.

- People who post messages may act as if they are knowledgeable about a topic, but they may know little or nothing about it.

Check out the following table for examples of e-mail lists.

Content Focus	List Name	Web Address
General fibromyalgia	Fibrom-L	www.fmscommunity.org/fibromhelp.htm
Guaifenesin	Guai-Support Group	www.netromall.com/guai-support
Fibromyalgia and chronic fatigue syndrome	Co-Cure (Cooperate and Communicate for a Cure)	www.co-cure.org/ccabout.htm

Noting newsgroups

A *newsgroup,* also known as a *Usenet group,* is an online special-interest group that usually doesn't require you to subscribe, fill out any forms, or agree to anything. You can read all the messages without ever making any public comments or revealing your presence. Or you can post messages and read replies. Some newsgroups are moderated by one or more people who set rules and make sure participants obey them. If not, they're warned and then may be thrown off. Many groups, however, aren't moderated, and it's a free-for-all kind of atmosphere. This can be good or bad, depending on your viewpoint.

Here are some of the good things about joining a newsgroup:

✔ Newsgroups often offer good or at least interesting information (as long as you read everything skeptically).

✔ Newsgroups give most readers strong moral support.

✔ Posters offer direct Web links to useful journal articles that you'd probably never find on your own.

When you find pros, you often find cons:

✔ Newsgroups are open to the world at large, and consequently, some people write obscene and/or ridiculous and insulting messages.

✔ Some individuals try to sell products, either overtly or covertly.

✔ People who aren't knowledgeable may offer cures or solutions that don't work or even exist.

Contact your Internet service provider to determine how to reach newsgroups. You can also find links to many newsgroups (including alt.med.fibromyalgia) at this Web site: www.makoa.org/usenet.htm.

Following forums

An online forum is a place where people with a special interest can usually find a great deal of information, read messages, and post their own messages. Forums are also known as message boards, discussion boards, or bulletin boards. At least one person usually moderates forums.

America Online (AOL) offers message boards about numerous topics, including fibromyalgia, chronic fatigue syndrome, and many others. AOL users can type **fibromyalgia** as a keyword to locate message groups and other sites available on AOL.

Often, topics, such as fibromyalgia, are subsumed under other topics. For example, on the About Arthritis forum, extensive information is provided on fibromyalgia at arthritis.tqn.com/msub15.htm. Go to this site and click on the subject links that fascinate you the most.

Pondering Publications

Several national newsletters or magazines are dedicated to fibromyalgia as of this writing. These publications include the following:

- ✔ *AFSA Update:* Published by the American Fibromyalgia Syndrome Association, Inc., 6380 E. Tanque Verde, Suite D, Tucson, AZ 85715; Phone: 520-733-1570; Internet: www.afsafund.org.

- ✔ *Fibromyalgia Aware:* Published by the National Fibromyalgia Association, 2238 N. Glassell Street, Suite D, Orange, CA 92865; Phone: 714-921-0150; Internet: www.fmaware.org.

- ✔ *Fibromyalgia Frontiers:* Published by the National Fibromyalgia Partnership, 140 Zinn Way, Linden, VA 22642-5609; Phone: 866-725-4404; Internet: www.fmpartnership.org.

- ✔ *Fibromyalgia Network:* Published Fibromyalgia Network, P.O. Box 31750, Tucson, AZ 85751; Phone: 800-853-2929; Internet: www.fmnetnews.com.

Index

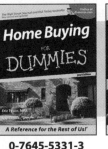
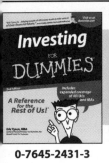
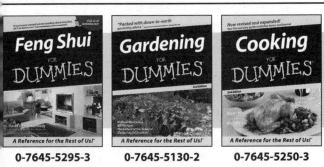
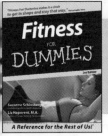
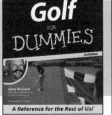
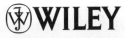

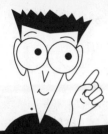
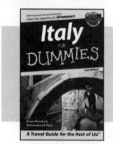
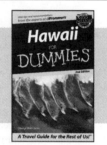
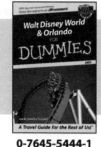
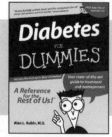
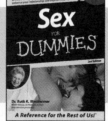
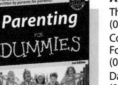

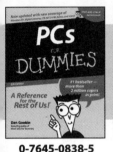
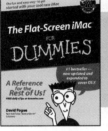
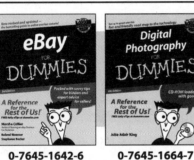
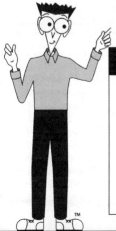

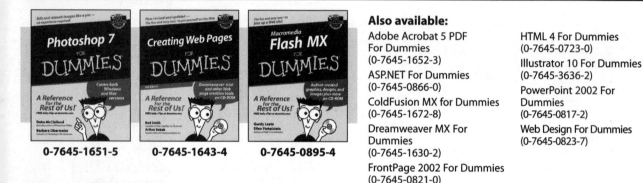
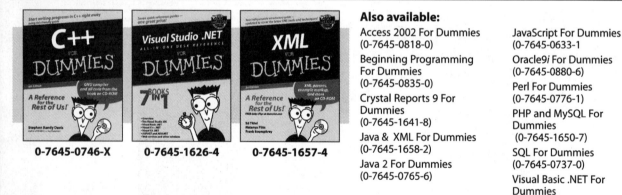
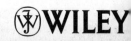

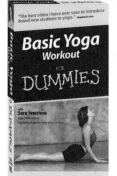
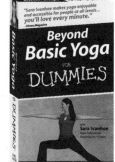
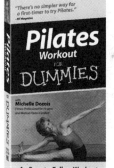
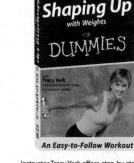
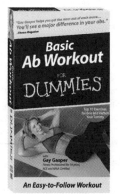
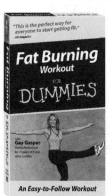
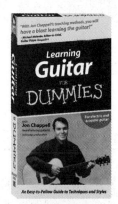